CONTENTS

ABOUT

Viva!Health is a pa... ...e registered charity Viva!. We monitor the scientific research linking diet to health and provide accurate information on which people can make informed choices about the food they eat.

We regularly communicate this information to the public, health professionals, schools and food manufacturers by:

- launching dynamic campaigns
- producing groundbreaking scientific reports
- publishing informative guides to help the public's understanding of health
- producing simple fact sheets on complex subjects
- regularly contributing to the highly-acclaimed *Viva!life* magazine
- running the Vegan Recipe Club with many tips and delicious recipes

DEFINITIONS

- OMNIVORE, MEAT-EATER – a person who eats everything, doesn't avoid any food groups
- SEMI-VEGETARIAN – a person who eats meat occasionally or avoids certain types of meat (eg red meat)
- PESCO-VEGETARIAN or PESCATERIAN – a person who doesn't eat meat but consumes fish and seafood
- VEGETARIAN – a person who eats no red meat, white meat, fish or seafood or slaughterhouse by-products such as gelatine, animal fat, lard or rennet
- VEGAN – a person who eats no animal products at all including meat, fish, seafood, milk and dairy products, eggs, honey and other food components derived from animals

VEGAN NUTRITION IN A NUTSHELL

A varied diet based on the foods in the table below ensures adequate intake of all essential nutrients and many more beneficial ones such as antioxidants. A healthy vegan diet is one consisting mainly of fruit and vegetables, pulses, wholegrains and nuts and seeds. It provides the body with all it needs and the only vitamin required to be supplemented is vitamin B12. It can be taken either in the form of food supplements or enriched foods, such as plant milks or margarines. B12 supplementation is not only recommended to vegans but to everyone over the age of 50, regardless of the diet, as the body's ability to absorb this vitamin declines with age.

Over the winter months, vitamin D supplementation is also recommended to everyone in the UK.

To ensure sufficient intake of essential omega-3 fats, natural sources should be made part of a daily diet – milled flaxseed (linseed) or hempseed and their oils for cold food preparation, rapeseed oil for cooking and some nuts and seeds as a healthy addition to meals – eg walnuts and chia seeds.

WHAT I NEED TO EAT EACH DAY

NO. OF SERVINGS	FOODS	HEALTHY PORTION SIZE	TO PROVIDE
At least **8**	**Fruits...** Apples, Pears, Peaches, Oranges, Kiwi fruit, Bananas, Raisins, Berries, etc Eaten whole or in smoothies (juices are more acidifying because they don't contain fibre and provide fruit sugar more readily than whole fruit) **And vegetables** Broccoli, Cauliflower, Spinach, Kale, Leeks, Carrots, Peppers, Tomatoes, Squash, Green beans, Sweet potatoes, Celery, Lettuce, Cabbage, Brussels sprouts, etc	**Fresh fruit**: 1 medium piece (the size of a tennis ball) **Dried fruit**: 1-1 ½ tablespoons or 1 golf ball **Green or root vegetables**: 2-3 tablespoons or ½ tennis ball **Salad vegetables**: 1 large cereal bowl or 80g	Folate (folic acid), Beta carotene, Vitamin C and other antioxidants, Fibre, Calcium, Iron
3-4	**Wholegrains** Millet, Quinoa, Brown and Wild rice, Spelt, Wheat, Buckwheat, Wholegrain bread, Muesli, Wholegrain pasta, etc	**Cooked grains**: 2-3 heaped tablespoons or ½ cup **Breakfast cereal**: 30g or 1 regular sized cereal bowl **Muesli**: 45g or a small sized bowl **Cooked wholemeal pasta**: 1 cup as side dish or 2 cups as main dish **Wholemeal or rye bread**: 2 slices	Energy, Fibre, B Vitamins, Calcium, Iron, Protein
3-4	**Pulses** Beans (pinto, white, butter, kidney, black-eyed, soya etc), Lentils, Peas, Chickpeas, Tofu and Soya and Bean products (burgers, sausages, mock meat, etc) **Nuts or seeds** Almonds, Brazil nuts, Cashew nuts, Pumpkin seeds, Sesame seeds, Flaxseed, etc	½ cup (cooked) 2 tablespoons	Protein, Energy, Fibre, Iron, Calcium, Other minerals
Small amounts	**Vegetable oil** Flaxseed, Hempseed oil, used cold; Olive oil or Rape seed oil for cooking Margarine	1 teaspoon per portion	Energy, Vitamin E (oils), Vitamin A & D (fortified margarine), Essential Omega-3 and Omega-6 Fats (flax seed, soya, walnut, hemp)
At least **1**	**B12 Fortified Foods** eg Fortified soya milk, Fortified breakfast cereal, Yeast extract (eg Marmite) Or B12 supplement		Vitamin B12

About **2** litres of water per day (at least eight glasses) should also be consumed as part of a healthy, balanced diet. Unsweetened hot beverages and natural juices can be counted as water.

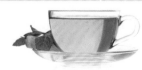

NUTRIENTS IN VEGAN DIET

NUTRIENT	FUNCTION	SOURCES
Protein	Vital for growth, development and repair of body tissues. Helps enzymes and hormones to function	Pulses (Peas, Beans, Lentils), Soya (eg Tofu, Soya Milk, Soya Mince), Wholegrains (eg Brown Rice), Cereals, Seeds & Seed Paste (eg Tahini), Beansprouts, Nuts (all types)
Fats	Carry some vitamins and energy to cells. Essential fats are vital to the brain, eyes and nerves and omega-3s are particularly anti-inflammatory	Seeds (esp. Linseed/Flaxseed), Hempseed and their oils, Dark Green Leafy Vegetables, Nuts & Nut Oils (esp. Walnuts), Tofu, Avocados, Olive Oil
Carbohydrates	Main source of energy	Wholegrains (Oats, Brown Bread, Brown Rice, Pasta eg Wholegrain Spaghetti, Rye), Potatoes, Sweet Potatoes, Beans, Peas & Lentils
Fibre	Keeps bowels healthy and regular; slows sugar and fat absorption and reduces cholesterol	Fruit & Vegetables, Wholegrains (Pasta, Brown Rice, Oats, Brown Bread), Nuts, Beans, Peas, Lentils
Vitamin A (Beta-Carotene)	Antioxidant. Vision, bone & teeth development, growth and tissue repair	Carrots, Sweet Potatoes, Red/Yellow Peppers, Tomatoes, Green Leafy Vegetables, Watercress, Mangoes, Apricots, Pumpkins, Cantaloupe Melons, Romaine Lettuce
B Group Vitamins B1 Thiamin, B2 Riboflavin, B3 Niacin, B5 Pantothenic Acid, B6 Pyridoxine, Folic Acid, Biotin	Absorption of energy, protein and fats, cell growth and nerve function	Brazil Nuts, Hazelnuts, Almonds, Green Leafy Vegetables, Brewers Yeast, Wholegrains, Beansprouts, Broad Beans, Bananas, Avocados, Mushrooms, Wheatgerm, Currants, Soya Mock Meats, Yeast Extract, Peanuts, Peas
Vitamin B12	Nerve formation, red blood cell production and allows us to use nutrients such as protein	Fortified products, including Soya Milks, Yeast Extract (eg Marmite), Breakfast Cereals and Margarines, Soya Mock Meats
Vitamin C	For healthy skin, teeth, bones and connective tissue. Aids iron absorption, important in disease resistance and for proper functioning of the immune system	Oranges, Grapefruit, Broccoli, Spinach, Cabbage, Blackcurrants, Strawberries, Green Peppers, Parsley, Potatoes, Peas
Vitamin D	Essential for the absorption of calcium and phosphate. (Sunlight enables the body to make Vitamin D in the skin.) Supports the immune system	Sunlight on the skin, Fortified Margarine, Fortified Breakfast Cereals, Fortified Soya Milk

NUTRIENT	FUNCTION	SOURCES
Vitamin E	Antioxidant. Helps protect the skin from UV damage; needed for lung membranes; stops fats in cell membranes going rancid	Vegetable Oils, Wheatgerm, Wholegrains, Tomatoes, Nuts (esp. Almonds), Sunflower and other Seeds, Avocados, Asparagus, Spinach, Apples, Carrots, Celery
Vitamin K	Essential for blood clotting. Half our requirements can be made by bacteria in the gut	Broccoli, Lettuce, Cabbage, Spinach, Brussel Sprouts, Asparagus
Calcium	Bone and teeth structure; muscle contractions; blood clotting and nervous system. Also vital to some hormones	Sesame Seeds and other Seeds, Pulses (Tofu from Soya, all types of Beans, Peas, Lentils), Broccoli, Watercress and other Green Leafy Veg, Swede, Almonds, Brazil Nuts, Fortified Soya Milk, Cinnamon, Fennel, Olives
Iron	Vital for red blood cell production to transport oxygen around the body and energy production	Beans, Lentils, Peas, Broccoli, Spinach, Cabbage, Wholegrains, Dried Apricots, Prunes, Figs, Dates, Pumpkin Seeds, Black Treacle, Cocoa, Turmeric, Thyme
Iodine	Makes thyroid hormones: vital for regulating metabolism	Green Leafy Vegetables, Asparagus, Sea Vegetables (eg Kelp), Vecon Vegetable Stock, Strawberries
Magnesium	Skeletal formation, metabolism, production of DNA, energy and muscle & nerve function	Green Leafy Vegetables, Nuts (eg Cashews, Almonds), Avocados, Wholegrains, Bananas, Apricots, Apples, Prunes
Potassium	Fluid balance, muscle & nerve impulse function, heart muscle function	Fennel, Brussel Sprouts, Broccoli, Aubergines, Cantaloupe Melons, Tomatoes, Parsley, Cucumber, Turmeric, Apricots, Ginger Root, Strawberries, Avocados, Bananas, Cauliflower, Cabbage, Almonds
Zinc	Involved in metabolism, wound healing and immunity. Also essential for healthy sperm, skin, taste and smell	Lentils, Peas, Beans (inc Tofu from Soya),Wholegrains (eg Rice, Bread etc), Green Leafy Veg, Nuts and Seeds (esp. Pumpkin Seeds), Brewers Yeast, Basil, Thyme
Others: Selenium, Cobalt, Copper, Manganese, Molybdenum	Dental, skeleton and skin health, hair and red blood cell growth and metabolism	Spinach, Broccoli, Peas, Beans, Lentils, Brewers Yeast, Almonds, Brazil Nuts, Bananas, Potatoes, Wholegrains, Seaweeds

For further information on nutrients in vegan diets, please see Viva!Health's guide *Nutrition in a Nutshell*: www.vivahealth.org.uk/resources/nutrition-nutshell.

VEGAN DIETS AND WORLD HEALTH INSTITUTIONS

In recent years, the popularity of veganism has risen sharply and many more people are now becoming vegan or buying vegan products than ever before. National and international health institutions pay close attention to all health and nutrition issues and have been producing studies and statements on plant-based diets for many years. The public is not always aware but the support for veganism from these institutions is overwhelming. Here's what they say about vegan diets:

American Dietetic Association (Craig & Mangels, ADA, 2009): "It is the position of the American Dietetic Association that appropriately planned vegetarian diets, including total vegetarian or vegan diets, are healthful, nutritionally adequate, and may provide health benefits in the prevention and treatment of certain diseases. Well-planned vegetarian diets are appropriate for individuals during all stages of the life cycle, including pregnancy, lactation, infancy, childhood, and adolescence, and for athletes."

British Dietetic Association (Garton, BDA, 2014): "Well planned vegetarian diets can be nutritious and healthy. They are associated with lower risks of heart disease, high blood pressure, type 2 diabetes, obesity, certain cancers and lower cholesterol levels."

British Nutrition Foundation (Philips, BNF, 2005): "In terms of nutrition, vegan and vegetarian diets can be nutritionally adequate, provided they are carefully planned."

Canadian Paediatric Society (Amit, CPS, 2010): "Well-planned vegetarian and vegan diets with appropriate attention to specific nutrient components can provide a healthy alternative lifestyle at all stages of foetal, infant, child and adolescent growth."

Food and Agriculture Organisation & World Health Organisation (2001): "Households should select predominantly plant-based diets rich in a variety of vegetables and fruits, pulses or legumes, and minimally processed starchy staple foods."

NUTRITION STATUS OF THE UK POPULATION

Latest results of an in-depth survey of nutrition status of the British population, The National Diet and Nutrition Survey, revealed that there's a lot of room for improvement (PHE & FSA, 2014).

The average intake of saturated fat, sugars and salt were above dietary recommendations while the intakes of fruit and vegetables and complex carbohydrates (such as wholegrains) were below. It's worth noticing that although the intake of the most health-detrimental fats, trans fats, was within the recommended limits, the main sources were milk and dairy products and meat and meat products (all these foods naturally contain trans fats). Trans (also called hydrogenated) fats increase blood cholesterol levels much more than saturated fat. Processed foods can contain these fats too but milk and meat contain them naturally.

When looking at vitamin intakes, teenage girls had low intakes of vitamin A, riboflavin (vitamin B2) and folate (vitamin B9). Older women were also found to have lower intakes of folate.

Vitamin D is a special category as it's the one vitamin our body produces when the skin is exposed to sunlight. The survey suggested there's an increased risk of vitamin D deficiency in all age/sex groups.

Mineral intakes vary but overall, the intake of iron was lower in teenage girls and older women and the survey also raised concerns that most people (including children) have lower than recommended intakes of magnesium, potassium, selenium and some other minerals.

All the above are easily corrected with a wholesome vegan diet, with the exception of vitamin D for which supplementation is now recommended for the entire population.

NUTRITION STATUS OF VEGETARIANS AND VEGANS

There are many recent studies analysing the diet composition and nutrient intakes of vegetarians and vegans from across the world.

In the most recent one, vegan, vegetarian, semi-vegetarian, pesco-vegetarian and omnivore diets were studied and compared in Belgium (Clarys et al., 2014). Vegans had the healthiest weight among all groups and received the highest score on the healthy eating scale (measured by two different ranking systems). The higher the score, the healthier the diet and the lower the risk of a number of chronic and lifestyle related diseases. The fat intake of the vegan group was better (more unsaturated healthy fats and less saturated fats) than in the other groups and they were also found to consume the most fibre and iron. Calcium intake was lower than in the other dietary patterns but still above the UK recommended dose (700 mg). Vegan protein intake was more than sufficient, whilst in meat eaters it reached almost twice the recommended intake levels, which has been shown to have negative health effects.

A similar study comparing various dietary patterns (omnivore, semi-vegetarian, pesco-vegetarian, lacto-ovo vegetarian and vegan) in the US and Canada brought similar results (Rizzo et al., 2013). Vegans had the healthiest body weights, the highest intake of fibre and the lowest fat intake. The overall fat intake of vegans was healthier than in the other groups – they ate the least saturated and trans fats. The vegan group was found to have more than sufficient intakes of protein, vitamins and minerals (including calcium and

iron above recommended intake). Based on the findings, the study authors suggested that the health protective effects of plant-based diets can be ascribed to the generally healthier profile of vegetarian diets.

When Davey et al. (2003) analysed food intakes of British vegans, vegetarians and meat-eaters, their findings were in line with the above. Vegans had the lowest intake of saturated fats and the highest intakes of fibre, vitamin B1, folate, vitamin C, vitamin E, magnesium and iron. The only mineral that was slightly below the recommended intake in some vegans was calcium but overall, vegans showed to have adequate intakes of all essential nutrients and had the healthiest fat intake profile (the least saturated and the most unsaturated fats). The healthfulness of vegan diets was also confirmed by a later study of UK population in which vegan diets had the best nutrient profiles of all diet groups, including the lowest fat and the highest fibre intakes (Key et al., 2014).

Orlich et al. (2014) looked at vegetarian and non-vegetarian diets more closely to assess the main differences. They found that vegans eat the most fruit, vegetables, soya and soya products, grains, pulses, nuts and seeds; and the least sweets, fizzy drinks, fried potatoes, refined cereals and added fats. Overall, vegetarian diets, and especially vegan ones, had much healthier patterns than omnivorous diets reflecting that plant-based diets are not based simply on exclusion of animal products but lead to a higher quality diet.

VEGAN CHILDREN

A vegan diet is healthful and suitable for adults and children alike. All parents need to ensure good nutrition for their children and vegan parents tend to be very well informed of their children's nutritional needs. As mentioned above, the American Dietetic Association is very supportive of a vegan diet for everyone, including children (Craig & Mangels, ADA, 2009): "Appropriately planned vegan, lacto-vegetarian, and lacto-ovo-vegetarian diets satisfy nutrient needs of infants, children, and adolescents and promote normal growth."

Their statement paper also points out that children raised on vegetarian diets have similar adult height and weight as those who became vegetarian later in life and that plant-based diets in childhood and adolescence can help establish lifelong healthy eating patterns. Vegetarian children and adolescents have lower intakes of cholesterol, saturated fat and total fat and higher intakes of fruits, vegetables and fibre than their peers.

The Canadian Paediatric Society agree that a well-planned vegan diet is adequate and healthy at all stages of foetal, infant, child and adolescent growth (Amit, CPS, 2010). And the British Nutrition Foundation reassures that UK vegetarian and vegan children's growth and development are within the normal range (Philips, BNF, 2005).

While Viva!Health supports the recommendation that infants should be exclusively breastfed for the first six months of their life, it's not always possible and many parents need to use a formula milk. There has been much debate about soya formula milks, the only vegan alternative to human breast milk. Many studies looked into the issue and the latest review and meta-analysis collated all available human data to provide a complete picture (Vandenplas et al., 2014). The paper concluded that all anthropometric patterns (size, growth, development), nutrient levels and bone mineral content of children fed soya formula were similar to those of children fed cow's milk formula or breastfed. There was no negative effect on reproductive and endocrine functions and immune and cognitive parameters were similar in all groups. The authors stated that "In conclusion, modern soya-based infant formulas are evidence-based safety options to feed children requiring them."

A paper on vegan infant nutrition summarised the main considerations for vegan parents (Mangels and Messina, 2001). The authors highlighted that appropriately planned vegan diets can satisfy nutrient needs of infants and that vegan babies show growth rates similar to other infants. They emphasised that breastfed vegan infants may need supplements of vitamin B 12 or that vegan mothers need to increase their B12 intake, older infants may need zinc supplements and good sources of iron and vitamins D and B12 – depending on their overall food intake.

The same scientific team also looked into vegan children's health (Messina and Mangels, 2001). Their review states that diets of vegan children meet or exceed recommendations for most nutrients and have higher intakes of fibre, lower intakes of fat, saturated fat and cholesterol than omnivore children. The only concerns the authors expressed was that some studies indicate vegan children have slightly lower calcium intakes.

However, with the growing number and availability of fortified foods suitable for vegans, it's now easy for children to meet all nutrient needs, including vitamins B12 and D.

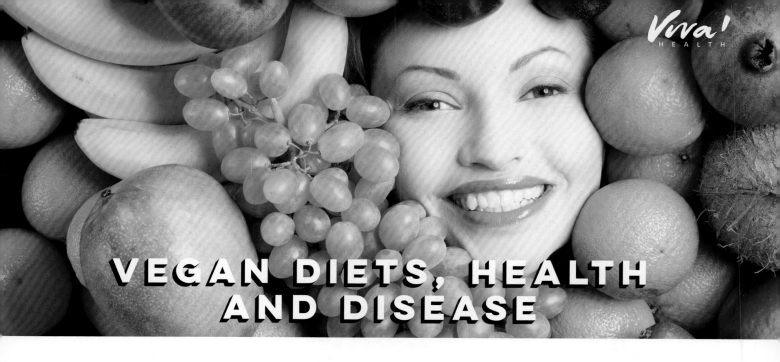

VEGAN DIETS, HEALTH AND DISEASE

VEGAN HEALTH AT A GLANCE

People who choose vegetarian or vegan diets often learn more about nutrition and the importance of various food groups and nutrients. As a result, they can make better food choices and tend to be more health conscious as demonstrated by Bedford and Barr (2005). A vegan diet is not necessarily a healthy one because many unhealthy, processed foods high in fat and sugar are also suitable for vegans, however vegan diets tend to be healthier and include more health-protective foods than omnivorous diets.

The studies above illustrate the quality and healthfulness of vegan diets but there is a wealth of research revealing much more. A 2010 review of the effects of vegan diets on health stated that compared with other vegetarian diets, vegan diets contain less saturated fat and cholesterol and more fibre (Craig, 2010). As a result, vegans tend to be slimmer, have lower blood cholesterol and blood pressure which reduces their risk of heart disease. Craig also mentioned that based on his research vegan diets have a cancer-protective effect and highlighted that vegans have a considerably higher intake of foods and nutrients protective against cancer.

Another review by Fraser (2009) pooled data from studies on vegetarian diets and health. Although he acknowledges that vegetarian diets can vary to a high degree, he says there is convincing evidence that vegetarians have lower rates of heart disease, low cholesterol levels, lower rates of hypertension and diabetes and lower prevalence of obesity. He also emphasised vegetarians' cancer rates are lower than those of others living in the same communities and

they have longer life expectancy. And Huang et al. (2012), who also reviewed scientific data on the subject, agree – vegetarians (including vegans) have increased longevity, lower risk of heart disease (and all risk factors for heart disease) and cancer.

One of the latest papers focusing specifically on the health of North American vegans brought interesting insights (Le and Sabaté, 2014). Compared to vegetarian diets (including dairy and eggs), vegan diets seem to offer greater protection from obesity, hypertension, type 2 diabetes and heart disease related mortality.

An exhaustive review of the literature published between 1950 and 2013 on chronic diet-related diseases such as obesity, diabetes, heart disease, kidney and liver disorders and cancers confirmed that plant food groups, especially unrefined plant-based foods, are more protective than animal food groups (Fardet and Boirie, 2014). Whilst plant-based diets contribute to good health, the authors warned that diets based on animal foods seriously increase the risk of chronic diseases.

Scientists agree that it's not simply avoidance of animal products that matters but that vegetarian and vegan diets' overall composition is what makes them healthier. Tuso et al. (2013) assert that plant-based diets are cost-effective, low-risk interventions that can reduce body weight, blood pressure, cholesterol levels and improve blood sugar control. The authors state that "They [plant-based diets] may also reduce the number of medications needed to treat chronic diseases and lower ischemic heart disease mortality rates. Physicians should consider recommending a plant-based diet to all their patients, especially those with high blood pressure, diabetes, cardiovascular disease, or obesity."

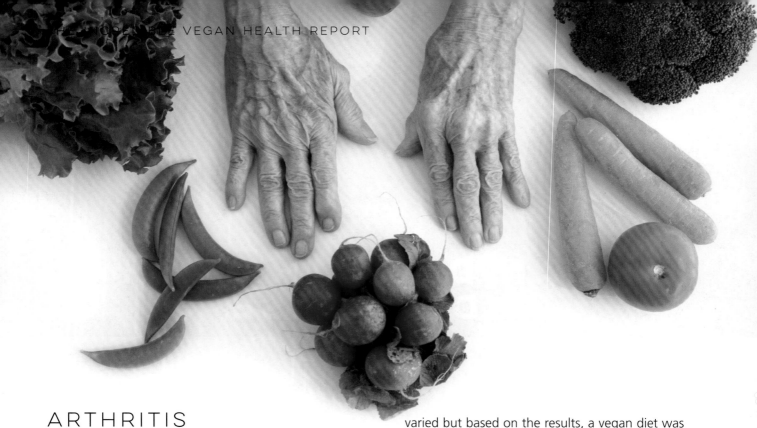

ARTHRITIS

Arthritis is the inflammation of joints. It causes joint pain and stiffness which usually worsens with age. The most common types of arthritis are osteoarthritis and rheumatoid arthritis.

Osteoarthritis causes the cartilage that covers joint surfaces to break down. Rheumatoid arthritis (RA) is an autoimmune disorder causing the immune system to attack the lining of joints and degrade it.

A vegan diet has been shown to be able to improve the health of RA sufferers and reduce the pain and stiffness of joints. Research revealed that people suffering from RA have inflammation of the intestinal tract resulting in increased permeability of the gut wall. With increased intestinal permeability, foreign proteins from foods and bacteria can pass into the bloodstream and cause an immune reaction that can harm joint lining. Fasting is known to decrease intestinal permeability and improve the symptoms of patients with RA but when patients return to a diet with dairy products the gut becomes more permeable and the arthritis returns (McDougall, 2002).

Several research teams have studied the impact of fasting followed by a vegan or vegetarian diet on patients with RA. Kjeldsen-Kragh's trial (1999) was the biggest one and it tested the effect of fasting for seven to 10 days, followed by three and a half months of an individually adjusted gluten-free vegan diet and for the next nine months consuming an individually adjusted vegetarian diet. Compared to the control group of RA patients who didn't change their diet, the diet change group improved significantly. The level of improvement

varied but based on the results, a vegan diet was recommended as a part of RA treatment. Müller *et al.* (2001) reviewed all available studies with a similar design and reached the conclusion that a vegan diet is more effective than vegetarian.

Hänninen *et al.* (2000) and Nenonen *et al.* (1998) studied the effects of a raw vegan diet on people with RA. These people volunteered to follow a diet of berries, fruits, vegetables and roots, nuts, germinated seeds and sprouts for three months. Their intake of antioxidants, fibre and health-protective phytochemicals increased significantly. In both studies, the rheumatoid patients who followed the diet for at least two months reported significant alleviation of their symptoms (joint pain, stiffness, swelling) but once they returned back to their omnivorous diet, the symptoms got worse.

Apart from the high intake of nutrients helping to improve health and decrease inflammation, the diets in the studies above also led to dramatic positive changes in the intestinal bacteria (Hänninen *et al.*, 2000; Kjeldsen-Kragh, 1999; Peltonen *et al.*, 1997). The bacteria species that thrive on plant-based foods are those that can significantly reduce inflammation and therefore the symptoms of arthritis. On the other hand, bacteria promoted by meat-based and fatty diets can increase the inflammation through toxic by-products of their metabolism. The study authors remarked that the greater the change in the gut microflora was, the better the patients' health was.

A recent review (Lahiri *et al.*, 2012) agreed that an antioxidant-rich diet can improve arthritis symptoms and can also help prevent the condition from developing. However, it's the overall diet that matters and the study highlighted that fruit and vegetable consumption is more important than supplements.

Hafström *et al.* (2001) tested the effects of a gluten-free vegan diet in an effort to eliminate gluten as a potential irritant. They assigned a group of RA sufferers to a diet consisting of fruit and vegetables, nuts, seeds and grains such as buckwheat, millet, corn and rice for one year and followed them throughout. Compared to the control group (who were following their usual, omnivorous diet), patients on the vegan diet achieved improvement in all clinical symptoms. The patients also had regular blood tests and in the vegan group, the levels of antibodies involved in the immune response to food irritants significantly decreased. This can be an important factor in decreasing joint inflammation.

Because dietary modifications have long been known to improve arthritis but fasting, gluten-free or a raw diet is not always possible or sustainable in the long term, Dr McDougall's team set out to test what they deemed to be an effective, inexpensive and practical dietary approach – a low-fat vegan diet (McDougall *et al.*, 2002). Plant-based foods consistently prove to be beneficial for people with arthritis but fats are known to have a negative effect so the diet had to be low in fat. They enlisted rheumatoid arthritis sufferers with moderate to severe degree of the illness who previously didn't follow a vegan or dairy-free diet. These patients were prescribed a wholesome, low-fat vegan diet for four weeks (based on pulses, wholegrains, fruit and vegetables). At the end of the test period, the participants lost on average three kilograms and their symptoms dramatically improved: pain and limitation in ability to function decreased and joint tenderness, swelling and severity of morning stiffness also decreased. Patients with the most active form of disease experienced the biggest improvements while patients with long-standing disease that had already destroyed most of the joint tissues experienced smaller improvements.

People with rheumatoid arthritis have an increased risk of cardiovascular disease. The fat levels in their blood tend to be higher and they have higher levels of cholesterol and LDL ('bad') cholesterol – both these patterns are related to inflammation. Elkan *et al.* (2008) focused on these issues when they tested the long-term effects (one year) of a gluten-free vegan diet as a dietary treatment for RA. The vegan group patients not only improved in terms of RA symptoms but their cholesterol levels improved and they lost weight – both

CASE STUDY: EMMA BRADLEY, REDDITCH

I have suffered from two main health problems during my life, rheumatoid arthritis and being overweight. The first, rheumatoid arthritis was diagnosed at just 18 months. I have spent much of my life taking drugs, attending physiotherapy and hydrotherapy just to stay mobile. During 'flare-up' periods I needed help even to get out of bed and yet at quiet periods I was able to walk reasonable distances and even take part in aerobics classes.

My other health problem was being overweight, this was partially due to restrictions in mobility but also poor nutrition. I became a vegetarian aged thirteen but replaced meat with cheese. Later on in my life, having my daughter made me really 'look' at our diet and change it to include plenty of fruit and vegetables. Going vegan was not as difficult as we thought it would be. We learnt to cook new things and found replacements for our favourite foods. A major benefit for me and totally unexpected has been the considerable reduction in pain from my arthritis, so much so that I no longer need any medication. It's fantastic but I can't help but feel annoyed that despite all medical evidence no doctor or specialist ever passed this information on to either myself or my parents. I had a happy childhood but there were things I missed out on – climbing trees, riding a bike – and I'm left with deformed joints. I can't help but wonder, would it have been a different story if I'd stopped having dairy as a child?

these results are very desirable and are known to be important in the prevention of cardiovascular disease.

Overall, the research is very supportive of a vegan diet as a part of RA treatment. Some people react better to a gluten-free vegan diet but the exclusion of animal derived foods seems to be more important. McDougall team's model of a low-fat wholesome vegan diet for RA sufferers (McDougall *et al.*, 2002) was very efficient in terms of health and symptom improvement and is affordable and sustainable in the long term for everyone.

THE INCREDIBLE VEGAN HEALTH REPORT

ASTHMA

Asthma is a respiratory condition characterised by attacks of spasms in the airways, which causes difficulty in breathing, wheezing, chest-tightness and breathlessness. The condition also causes inflammation of the airways. The attacks are usually triggered by allergens or chemicals and diet can play an important role.

Dietary modifications have been shown to reduce the frequency or severity of the attacks. Although there aren't any studies of vegan diets and asthma, there is evidence that a diet based on plant foods and rich in fruit and vegetables can be very beneficial to asthma sufferers. Seyedrezazadeh et al. (2014) reviewed scientific studies examining the relationship between fruit and vegetable consumption and the risk of wheezing and asthma (in children and adults). They found out that people of all ages in the highest total fruit and vegetable intake category had a 36 per cent lower risk of asthma than people in the lowest intake categories. Overall, the results showed that low intake of fruit and vegetables was associated with an

increased risk of wheezing and asthma. The authors suggested that the high antioxidant content of these foods can play a role in preventing or reducing the airway inflammation.

Nagel et al. (2010) conducted a global study of diet and childhood asthma that involved 20 countries. Fruit, vegetable and fish intake was linked to a lower risk of asthma and wheeze. However, the fish intake is debatable because fish are a source of polyunsaturated (omega-3) fats and the study didn't follow the other sources of these fats such as nuts and seeds and pulses which would have made it possible to compare the effect of the different sources of these fats. On the other hand, the results showed that meat and burger intake in particular, was associated with an increased risk of asthma.

Rodríguez-Rodríguez et al. (2014) wanted to explore the possible link between dietary fats and asthma in children so they conducted a large study of eight to 13 year old schoolchildren. They found out that diets

---

CASE STUDY: JAY, 43, CORNWALL

In my late thirties I began to get wheezy and chesty. I also had a near-constant cold. I was prescribed a brown 'preventer' inhaler and a blue 'reliever' inhaler, both of which I used regularly.

I always considered myself to be fit; I had run regularly during my twenties, a few injuries and niggles meant that I slowed down in my thirties but I still hiked, walked the dogs, etc., and so thought I was quite active. My wife and I had been vegetarian for years then but she made the decision to go vegan. I'll admit that I wasn't very supportive initially, I didn't understand veganism and why she wanted to do something so 'extreme'.

She didn't try to influence me, knowing that it would likely have the opposite effect, but I ate all of the meals she cooked and so my dairy intake naturally decreased. I also glanced at the odd Viva!life magazine strategically placed around the house. I then came across a series of books about long-distance running: Born To Run *by Christopher McDougall,* Eat & Run *by Scott Jurek, and* Finding

Ultra *by Rich Roll. Suddenly a vegan diet wouldn't just allow me to run; it would help me to run.*

Everything quickly came together – an understanding of the animal ethics, an understanding of the environmental impact I was still having, the happy realisation that far from having a restricted diet we were eating better food than we had in years, and the knowledge that this could all support me to get back to running. That was three years ago. I started slow, one mile – three miles – five miles, a 10k. After a year I was doing half marathon distances. In April this year I ran the Paris marathon with my wife (her first marathon and she couldn't run a mile the previous year), in May I ran the Classic Quarter in Cornwall – 44 miles around the hilly coastal path. I have just signed up for the Transvulcania ultramarathon – a 74km run with a 8028m accumulated elevation. My goal is to eventually run the 170km Ultra-Trail Du Mont-Blanc.

I haven't used my inhalers at all since around six months after becoming vegan! I don't consider myself to have asthma any more.

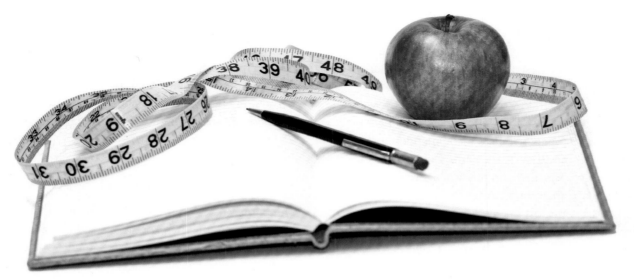

higher in fat, and saturated fat in particular, were linked to asthma. The main source of these in the children's diet was butter and the asthma sufferers also had higher intake of dairy products in general.

In terms of asthma control, regular consumption of raw vegetables was shown to be very beneficial by Iikura *et al.* (2013). They examined over 400 long-term asthma sufferers and their lifestyles. The common feature of people who had good control over their condition was routine intake of fresh vegetables and regular exercise.

In conclusion, fruit and vegetables consistently prove to be beneficial in asthma prevention and treatment, whilst animal foods have been found to be linked to an increased risk of asthma and to poorer asthma management.

BODY WEIGHT

Many studies compare dietary patterns in terms of their nutrient profile and healthfulness but also with respect to their effect on body weight. It's been shown time and again that vegan diets lead to healthy body weight even without portion restriction and they are the most effective in long-term weight management. Being overweight or obese is associated with hyperlipidemia (increased fat levels in the blood), hypertension, diabetes, cardiovascular disease, certain cancers and all-cause mortality so a healthy weight is a key factor in overall good health.

Berkow & Barnard (2006) reviewed all available studies on vegetarian diets and body weight and found that the majority of them reported a significantly lower body weight (four to 20 per cent) in vegetarians compared to non-vegetarians.

A large study of women and their dietary patterns (Newby *et al.*, 2005) reported that the prevalence of being overweight or obese among vegetarians is significantly lower than among omnivores. They highlighted that, in general, women eating plant-based diets have a much lower risk of becoming overweight or obese in the long term with vegans being at the lowest risk. The study also confirmed that vegans have the highest intake of fruit and vegetables and healthy carbohydrates (wholegrains, pulses and fibre).

The reason vegan diets work so well in terms of healthy weight maintenance is that they are lower in fat, have a better fat intake profile (less saturated and more essential unsaturated fats), lead to a higher intake of fibre and nutrient-rich foods and lower calorie intake (Berkow & Barnard, 2006; Huang *et al.*, 2015). People consuming low-fat carbohydrate-rich diets can eat more food in weight compared to others because these foods have lower energy density.

It's been well documented that vegans tend to have healthy weight, are at the least risk of being overweight but also do not tend to be underweight. When Tonstad *et al.* (2009) examined the relationship between different types of diet and body weight, they found that vegans were the only group who had a healthy BMI (body mass index – a ratio of body height and weight), whilst vegetarians, pesco-vegetarians and omnivores were all in the overweight category. The same conclusion was also reached in a later study of dietary patterns, health and cancer incidence (Tantamango-Bartley *et al.*, 2013).

To explore how a change of diet affects people who previously didn't follow a plant-based diet, Turner McGrievy *et al.* (2015) compared the effects of five different diets over the period of six months on participants' body weight. They assigned volunteers who were all overweight to one of the five groups – vegan, vegetarian, pesco-vegetarian, semi-vegetarian and omnivore. All were advised to eat a low-fat diet based on foods with low glycemic index (foods with low proportion of fast absorbing sugars) but there was no restriction on energy intake recommended to any of the groups in the study. Participants were free to eat until they were satisfied and physical activity did not differ between the groups. After six months, the vegan group participants lost on average 7.5 per cent of body weight, vegetarians 6.3, pesco- and semi-vegetarians lost 3.2 and omnivores 3.1 per cent. Based on the final analysis of the participants' diets, the vegan group had the lowest intake of fat in general, and saturated fat specifically, and the highest intake of carbohydrates and fibre. Also their cholesterol levels dropped significantly more than in any other group.

Huang et al. (2015) reviewed other intervention studies where people were prescribed a diet change and reached a similar conclusion as the study above. Individuals assigned to the vegetarian diet groups lost significantly more weight than those assigned to the non-vegetarian diet. A more detailed analysis revealed that vegan groups lost more weight than vegetarian ones. The study authors also remarked on the healthfulness of plant-based diets and their higher nutritional quality compared to other diets.

To investigate what a low-fat vegan diet can achieve in people who are overweight and/or have diabetes, Mishra et al. (2013) enlisted people on a trial that involved workplace cafeterias offering low-fat vegan options. The participants were instructed to eat a wholesome vegan diet low in fat for 18 weeks with no other changes to their daily life. Again, there were no portion or energy intake restrictions.

At the end of the 18 week study, the volunteers lost on average 4.3 kg, their cholesterol levels decreased dramatically and their blood sugar control improved. No significant differences were achieved by the control group (people who didn't change their diet or lifestyle but fulfilled the same criteria as the intervention group).

All these studies clearly show that a low-fat vegan diet can help achieve and maintain healthy weight without portion restriction and in the long-term. Many experts also recommend plant-based diets as a healthy, nutrient dense approach to weight management and prevention of obesity for adults and children alike (Farmer et al., 2011; Sabaté & Wien, 2010).

BONE HEALTH

The human body is a fine-tuned organism that works best only under certain conditions and is very sensitive to any changes in the inner environment. One of the most important characteristics of the body is a stable acid-alkali balance in the blood. The body neutralises any excesses of either acid or alkali to protect this vital balance but if there is too much acid, other systems in the body, such as the skeleton, can suffer. If there's too much acid, and calcium from the diet isn't enough to neutralise it, the body needs to draw on its calcium reserves in the muscles and bones. Some of the calcium is then deposited back to the bones but most of it is excreted in the urine together with the acids.

Diet influences the acid–alkali balance in the body and dietary data can be used as an estimate for endogenous acid production – ie the amount of acid produced in the body as a result of the food eaten. Some dietary factors contribute to dietary acid load more than others. Sulphur from sulphur amino acids (protein building blocks) is the main contributor because it is metabolised into sulphuric acid. Sulphur amino acids are highest in animal protein and therefore diets high in animal protein are likely to produce considerable amounts of acid in the body. Another contributor is phosphorus, which is mainly supplied by meat and dairy products. Potassium and magnesium, abundant in plant foods, and calcium, found in plant foods and dairy products, are determinants of alkaline load (Alexy et al., 2007).

A large, seven-year study of 1,035 women found that women with diets high in animal and low in plant protein had an almost four times higher rate of bone loss and their risk of hip fracture was 3.7 times that of women who consumed the least animal protein (Sellmeyer

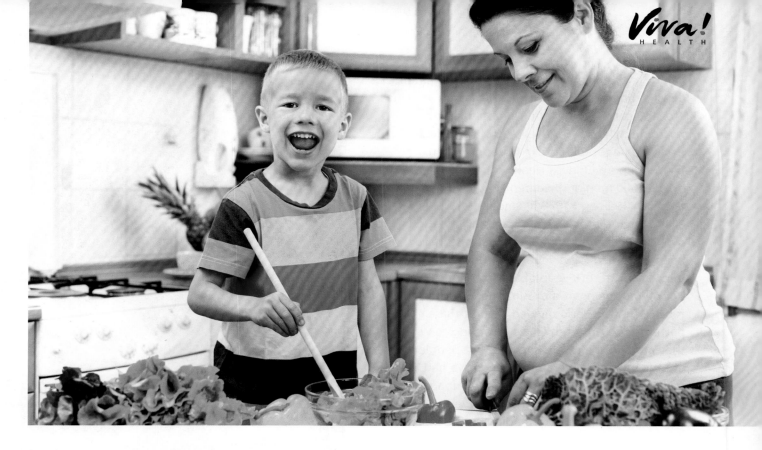

et al., 2001). Findings from another large study of women also showed a clear division – high intake of animal protein caused bone loss while high intake of vegetable protein did not and even contributed to increased bone density (Weikert et al., 2005).

Adequate calcium intake is important but it's the overall diet that matters. It is a known fact that countries with the highest calcium and animal protein intakes also have the highest fracture rates. The World Health Organization calls this calcium paradox and states: "The paradox (that hip fracture rates are higher in developed countries where calcium intake is higher than in developing countries where calcium intake is lower) clearly calls for an explanation. To date, the accumulated data indicate that the adverse effect of protein, in particular animal (but not vegetable) protein, might outweigh the positive effect of calcium intake on calcium balance." (WHO/FAO, 2003)

A large-scale study on calcium intake and bone health found that calcium intake above 750 mg a day didn't offer any protection from fractures and high calcium intakes increased the risk of hip fractures (Warensjö et al., 2011). This study involved over 60,000 women whose diets and health were followed for up to 19 years.

The UK recommended daily intake of calcium is 700 mg for adults and the latest studies revealed that vegans get enough calcium from their diet to meet this recommendation. See chapter Nutrition Status of Vegetarians and Vegans for more information.

An extensive review by Lanou (2009) resulted in a conclusion that: "bones are better served by attending to calcium balance and focusing efforts on increasing fruit and vegetable intakes, limiting animal protein, exercising regularly, getting adequate sunshine or supplemental vitamin D, and getting 500 mg calcium a day from plant sources."

A number of studies investigating the impact of diet on bone health have demonstrated the beneficial effect of fruit and vegetables on bone mass and bone metabolism in men and women across all age ranges. For example:

- Adolescent girls consuming more than three servings of fruit and vegetables had healthier and better bones and were losing less calcium in urine than girls consuming less (Tylavsky et al., 2004).
- A population-based study examined the association between fruit and vegetables intake and bone mineral density in 670 postmenopausal Chinese women (Chen et al., 2006). Analyses showed that high intake of fruit and vegetables was significantly associated with greater bone density at all locations measured.
- A project based at Human Nutrition Research, Cambridge, UK analysed a series of studies examining the association between fruit and vegetable consumption and bone mineral density (Ashwell et al., 2008). Significant associations were observed between bone

health markers (measurements of bone mineral density, bone resorption, loss of calcium in urine etc) and carotenoids (plant pigments) and vitamin E which suggested a positive effect of fruit and vegetable intake on bone health.

- The Singapore Chinese Health Study enrolled over 63,000 men and women aged 45-74 years between 1993 and 1998 in Singapore (Dai et al., 2014). Their diet has been repeatedly assessed over the years and two dietary patterns have been identified – the vegetable-fruit-soya pattern (mostly cruciferous vegetables, fruit and tofu items) and the meat-dim-sum (meat, processed food). The study also divided each of these patterns into different levels according to what they ate and the results showed that people who ate the most fruit, vegetables and soya had a 34 per cent lower risk of hip fracture compared to people who ate the least. The observed relationship appeared to be direct – the more of the healthy, plant-based foods people ate, the lower their risk of fracture and vice versa.

- The journal *Osteoporosis International* published a review of studies on bone health and acid-alkali balance in the body (Lambert et al., 2015). This review looked at studies where people were given alkaline salts (that naturally occur in fruit and vegetables) to supplement their diet and analysed the results. The researchers found that increasing the intake of alkalis meant reduced losses of calcium through urine and lower rate of bone degradation. They concluded that potassium salts (alkalis) have the potential to prevent osteoporosis and recommend an increased consumption of fruit and vegetables as a means to improve bone health (fruit and vegetables contain potassium and create alkalis during digestion).

A very interesting study of over 150 vegans looked at their diets in relation to bone health (Ströhle et al., 2011). The researchers evaluated participants' diets individually in terms of their acidifying or alkalising effect on the body. They used two models to work this out to be more precise. The results, regardless of the model used, revealed that vegan diets are characterised by a virtually neutral acid-alkali balance which is very desirable. Calcium intake in vegans was more than 800 mg which is above UK recommendation but lower than in average omnivores. The study authors suggested that given the fact that the low acidifying effect of vegan diets lowers urinary calcium loss, vegans may require less calcium than omnivore adults. In addition, higher

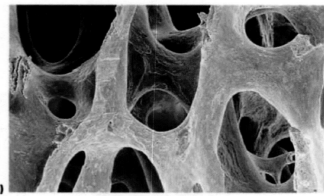

(a) Normal bone

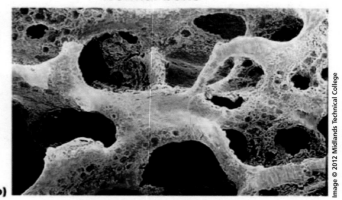

(b) Osteoporotic bone

Image © 2012 Midlands Technical College

phosphate intake is associated with increased calcium retention and the phosphate content of vegan diets could result in lower calcium requirements in vegans.

Ho-Pham et al. (2012) tested bone mineral density of vegan Buddhist nuns and omnivores, their fracture incidence and closely examined their diet. The results were very reassuring – over the two-year study period, vegans maintained bone mineral density much better than omnivores. With age, bone mineral density naturally decreases but omnivores in this study had twice the bone loss of vegans. The study also showed that low body weight, higher intakes of animal protein and fats and corticosteroid use were associated with greater rates of bone loss. What was of specific interest was that calcium intake of the study participants was relatively low, but it did not have adverse effect on bone loss. Indeed, the average dietary calcium intake among the vegan nuns was only 375 mg a day whilst the intake in non-vegetarians was 683 mg, and yet, based on the results, the vegans had better bone health.

There's plenty of evidence now that a vegan diet not only provides sufficient calcium but that it also ensures the intake of many bone-beneficial nutrients and minimises the potential damage to bones caused by dietary acid load.

CANCER

Cancer is a major threat to our health today but diet and lifestyle can significantly reduce or increase the risk of cancer in general and even more so for some types of cancer. In the UK, the lifetime risk of cancer has been on the rise for decades. Ahmad *et al.* (2015) estimated the risk of cancer for people of different ages based on past and current cancer rates and trends. The lifetime risk of cancer in the UK increased from 38.5 per cent for men born in 1930 to 53.5 per cent for men born in 1960. For women it increased from 36.7 to 47.5 per cent. For people born since 1960, the risk is 50 per cent. This means over half of people who are currently adults under the age of 65 years will be diagnosed with cancer at some point in their lifetime. Intimidating as this sounds, there are volumes of scientific studies showing a diet change can achieve a lot in terms of both prevention and treatment of cancer. There are thousands of studies linking diet to cancer so the below is a careful selection outlining the bigger picture.

World Cancer Research Fund and The American Institute for Cancer Research (2009) outline the most important preventable causes of cancer: smoking, unhealthy diets, physical inactivity and excess body weight. The report states that "the prevention of cancer is now one of the most important, achievable and potentially rewarding global public health challenges". It goes on to say that diets high in plant foods, and specifically non-starchy vegetables, fruits and other foods high in dietary fibre, vitamin C and carotenoids can protect against a number of cancers.

The report of World Cancer Research Fund and The American Institute for Cancer Research preceding the above document (2007) takes an in-depth look at diet, lifestyle and all relevant factors important in cancer prevention. One of the report's main recommendations is for people to eat mostly foods of plant origin, non-starchy vegetables (eg green leafy vegetables, cucumbers, peppers) and fruit consumption to be at least 600 grams daily (at least five portions) and wholegrains and/or pulses to be a part of every meal.

A recent study by Oxford University, looking at how diet affects cancer risk, revealed that vegans have a much lower risk of getting the disease (Key *et al.*, 2014). The 15-year-long study followed 60,000 British men and women, of which over 18,000 were vegetarians and 2,246 vegan. They found that overall cancer incidence (compared to meat-eaters) was 11 per cent lower in vegetarians and 19 per cent lower in vegans. This result corresponds with a review by Huang *et al.* (2012) that reached the conclusion that vegetarians (all groups of vegetarians together) have 18 per cent lower cancer rates than meat-eaters.

Another large study of almost 70,000 people, their dietary patterns and cancer incidence suggests that vegan diets are associated with a lower risk of all cancers combined and particularly with lower risk of female-specific cancers when compared with non-vegetarians (Tantamango-Bartley *et al.*, 2013). Vegetarians as a combined group had lower risk of all cancers and gastrointestinal cancers in particular than meat-eaters.

The well-known Cornell-Oxford-China Study, 'The China Study', conducted in the 1970s and 1980s demonstrated important relationships between dietary patterns and cancer risk (Campbell and Junshi, 1994). The study involved 65 Chinese counties and focused on their diets and health. Campbell and Junshi reported that several major diseases such as brain, breast, colon and lung cancer, leukemia, cardiovascular disease and diabetes were all associated with affluent diets. In other words, these diseases were directly associated with the intake of milk, meat, eggs, animal fat and protein whilst diets high in fibre, antioxidants (mainly from fruit and vegetables) and pulses seemed to have a preventative effect.

Authors of a comprehensive review of studies on cancer and diet (Lanou and Svenson, 2010) agree that diets rich in plant foods decrease the risk of many types of cancer. They point out that specific beneficial effects have been shown for fibre, fruits and vegetables, pulses including soya foods, seeds, spices and wholegrains.

Science also picked up on the anti-cancerous effects of cruciferous vegetables (broccoli, cabbage, radish, watercress, rocket). Abdull Razis and Noor (2013) decided to recapitulate the facts and investigate more closely why broccoli and other cruciferous species appear to have a strong preventative effect against many types of cancer (mostly colorectal, lung, prostate and breast). Cruciferous vegetables contain substantial amounts of glucosinolates, a class of sulphur-containing glycosides, and their breakdown products such as the isothiocyanates are believed to be responsible for their health benefits. This study found that both glucosinolates and isothiocyanates can modulate the activity of enzymes that are crucial for cancer-prevention.

Bosetti et al. (2012) analysed data from a series of studies from Italy and Switzerland and found that consumption of cruciferous vegetables at least once a week significantly reduced the risk of cancer of the oral cavity and pharynx, esophagus, colon and rectum, breast and kidney.

At the other end of the spectrum, diets based on animal products are known to present a risk in terms of cancer. Grant (2013) undertook a comprehensive study and analysed high-quality data from 87 countries to examine the relationship between lifestyle and cancer. The results showed that the main factor notably contributing to 12 types of cancer across the countries was animal product consumption (which included meat, milk, fish and eggs). The types of cancer that animal products were most strongly linked to were breast, uterus, kidney, ovarian, pancreatic, prostate, testicular and thyroid cancer and multiple myeloma. The study also documented how the rise of animal products consumption in some countries was followed by increased cancer rates. Examples of this include colon cancer rising after 15-27 years and breast cancer after

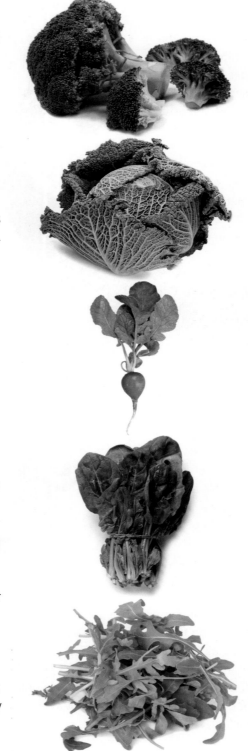

20-31 years in Japan and mortality rates for some cancers in several Southeast Asian countries increased 10 years after meat and dairy consumption rose. The author explained that animal product consumption causes increased production of insulin, insulin-like growth factor 1 and sex hormones in the body which is probably why it's so strongly linked to cancer. Higher levels of these hormones are known to increase the cancer risk for several organ systems (see next chapter for more details). Grant also pointed out that haem-iron in meat (this type of iron is only found in meat) may be a risk factor for cancer through increased production of free radicals and DNA damage. Furthermore, higher protein intake has been shown to stimulate cancer promoting reactions in the body and it was suggested that the only diet that could avoid these is a wholesome vegan diet excluding protein isolates.

The World Health Organisation (WHO), based on extensive research by its advisory body – The International Agency for Research on Cancer – recently classified processed meat as carcinogenic and red meat as probably carcinogenic (Bouvard et al., 2015).

It's been known for a long time that cooking meat at high temperatures produces carcinogenic compounds called polycyclic aromatic hydrocarbons (PAH) and heterocyclic amines. A recent study revealed that these compounds increase their carcinogenic potential when they chemically interact with nitrogen (a basic element in protein) and become nitrated (Jariyasopit et al., 2014). The study showed nitrated PAHs have six to 432 times higher potential to cause mutations, that can lead to cancer, than the parent compounds. High-temperature cooking of meat therefore poses a much bigger health risk than previously thought.

The most abundant of heterocyclic amines, a compound called PhiP, also has strong estrogenic effects and has been linked to hormone-sensitive cancers (Papaioannou *et al.*, 2014).

Some substances added to processed meat, such as nitrites used as preservatives, can also lead to the formation of carcinogenic N-nitroso compounds and these, together with an increased presence of PAHs (due to high temperature processing) and high content of haem-iron, might be the reason why processed meat has been shown to be more carcinogenic than red meat.

And another factor increasing the potential of animal-based foods to contribute to cancer are environmental pollutants such as polychlorinated biphenyls (PCBs). Although these industrial compounds were banned worldwide more than 30 years ago because of their high toxicity, they are very persistent and therefore still present in our environment. Once in the body, PCBs accumulate in the fat tissue and can cause long-term problems such as compromised immune response, mental and behavioural problems, decreased activity of the thyroid, reproductive problems, can induce cancer and severely damage the development of a baby. A review published in the journal *Environmental Medicine* revealed that in the food chain fish, dairy, hamburgers and poultry are the most contaminated foods (Crinnion, 2011).

IGF-1, DIET AND CANCER

Insulin-like Growth Factor 1 (IGF-1) is a hormone with a similar molecular structure to insulin. It's vital to childhood growth and encourages cell growth and proliferation in adults. It's naturally produced by the liver and its production is stimulated by growth hormones. The levels of IGF-1 are highest in childhood and decline in adulthood. However, IGF-1 also promotes each of the key stages of cancer development: growth of the cancerous cells, vascularisation of cancerous tissue (blood vessel growth) and metastasis. In addition, it also prevents natural cell death (apoptosis) so the effect on cells with cancer potential can be dramatic.

This influence, when applied to a large number of 'at risk' cells over many years, could ensure survival of these cells and accelerate carcinogenesis (Jenkins *et al.*, 2006).

Melnik *et al.* (2011) offers a valuable insight into this issue. As both insulin and IGF-1 are growth stimulators, any food or drink that stimulates the production of these two hormones is potentially health-detrimental. Milk and dairy products contain whey proteins which cause a rise in insulin, IGF-1 and growth hormone levels and as the authors explain, a typical Western diet rich in dairy and sugar (that also stimulates insulin production) shifts growth hormone and IGF-1 balance to abnormally high levels.

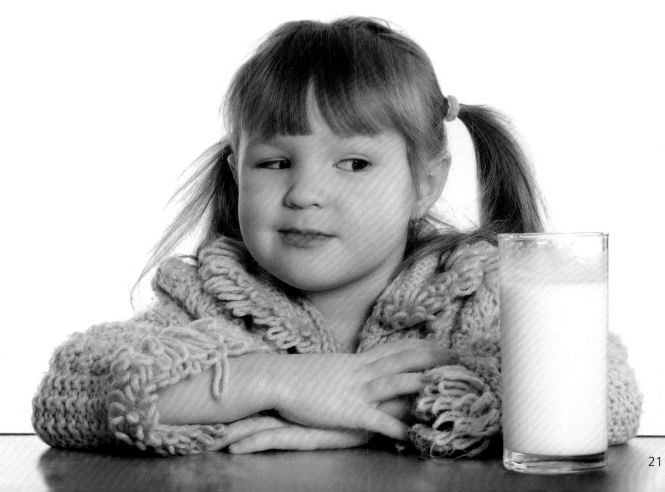

An analysis by Barnard (2004) is in agreement with the above and adds that the typical Western diet also contains a variety of mutagens and carcinogens that may increase the generation of oxygen radicals and lead to the initiation of cancer as well as other degenerative diseases. Barnard highlights the link between diet, lifestyle and increased levels of IGF-1, insulin and growth hormone. He suggests that a diet high in wholegrains, pulses, fruits and vegetables not only normalises the levels of these hormones but also contains large amounts of natural antioxidants that can prevent free radical formation and reduce oxidative stress in the body.

Vegan diets are associated with lower levels of IGF-1 and higher levels of IGF-binding proteins 1 and 2 (these proteins limit the availability of IGF-1) compared with an omnivorous or even a vegetarian diet (Tantamango-Bartley et al., 2013). As a part of the EPIC (The European Prospective Investigation into Cancer and Nutrition) study, Allen et al. (2000 and 2002) measured circulating levels of IGF-1 of British meat-eaters, vegetarians and vegans. Compared with meat-eaters and vegetarians, vegan women had 13 per cent lower levels of IGF-1 and the concentrations of both IGF-binding proteins 1 and 2 were 20–40 per cent higher. Vegan men had IGF-1 levels nine per cent lower than others and this difference was considered enough to significantly lower the risk of prostate cancer. The intake of animal protein was linked with elevated IGF-1 levels and diet explained most of the differences in IGF-1 concentration between the groups.

As milk and dairy products consumption has been suggested to play a role in the development of some types of cancer, Swedish scientists decided to do a population study and investigate whether lactose intolerant people get less cancer (Ji et al., 2015). The cancer types in question were lung, breast and ovarian. The researchers identified nearly 23,000 lactose intolerant people through health registers and compared their lung, breast and ovarian cancer incidence with that of the general population. And the results showed their predictions were correct – the risk of lung cancer was 45 per cent lower, breast cancer 21 per cent lower and ovarian cancer 39 per cent lower in lactose-intolerant individuals. The study also looked at cancer incidence in close family members of the study participants but their cancer rates were the same as in the general population. The authors of the study suggested that dairy products might be increasing cancer risk due to the high amounts of fats, particularly saturated fat, and some growth hormones, such as IGF-1 (both of which have been linked to the development of cancer).

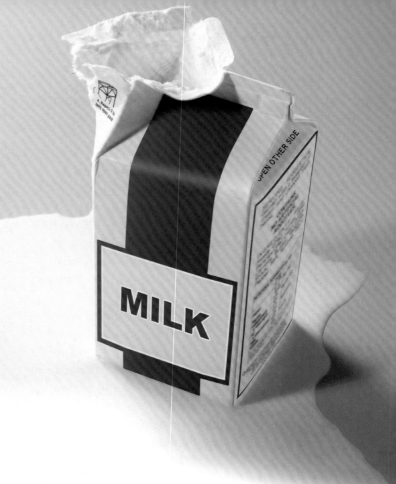

Almost all body cells respond to IGF-1 and diets increasing its levels are not only dangerous in terms of facilitating cancer growth but can have grave consequences in the case of hormone-sensitive cancers. Eliminating animal protein from the diet naturally decreases IGF-1 levels and therefore lowers the risk of cancer.

BREAST CANCER

Breast cancer has been at the scientists' centre of attention for many decades. It's not only one of the most frequent types of cancer but it can be hormone sensitive which makes the treatment more difficult. Diet has been linked not only to the prevention and treatment of breast cancer but also to natural regulation of hormone levels. In the case of breast cancer, diet is of high importance both because of nutrient content and due to its effect on body weight. Being overweight is one of the risk factors for breast cancer.

During the Shanghai Breast Cancer Study (Cui et al., 2007), a wealth of data from breast cancer patients and healthy women of similar age was collected and the risk of breast cancer in relation to diet evaluated. The authors noticed there were two dietary patterns – 'vegetable-soya', characterised by fruit and vegetables, pulses and grains; and 'meat-sweets' characterised by meat, fatty foods and sweets. The analyses of the data revealed that the 'meat-sweet' pattern was significantly associated with increased risk of estrogen receptor-positive breast cancer among postmenopausal women and this association was even stronger if the women were overweight.

Another large study was conducted in Singapore where 34,000 women's dietary patterns and health were followed for the average period of ten years (Butler *et al.*, 2010). Similar to the study above, the researchers identified two dietary patterns, 'meat-dim sum' and 'vegetable-fruit-soya'. And the results revealed a direct relationship between diet and breast cancer risk in postmenopausal women – the greater the intake of the foods from the vegetable-fruit-soya category, the lower the risk of breast cancer. More specifically, the risk was 30 per cent lower in women who had the highest intake of these foods.

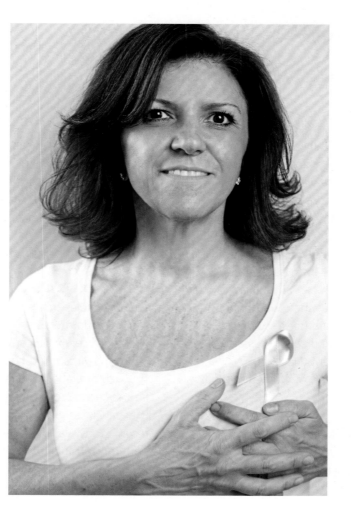

And when a long-term study followed women's health and diets in Italy, it arrived at a comparable conclusion (Sieri *et al.*, 2004). Women with mostly plant-based diets high in raw vegetables had up to 36 per cent lower risk of cancer than women who ate more animal-based and processed foods. The risk reduction was even higher for women who maintained a healthy weight.

Brennan *et al.* (2010) reviewed a myriad of studies on dietary patterns and breast cancer risk and reached a foreseeable conclusion – women consuming a diet high in plant-based foods, healthy fats and low in alcohol have a lower risk of breast cancer than women eating typical Western diets high in meat and animal fats.

As a part of the enormous Nurses' Health Study, a Harvard scientific team investigated whether there is any link between the risk of breast cancer and dietary protein source (Farvid *et al.*, 2014). During the 20 years of follow-up, it emerged that a higher intake of red meat was associated with an increased risk of breast cancer. When the effects of different protein sources were estimated based on the dietary data, the scientists arrived at the conclusion that substituting one serving a day of red meat for one serving of pulses would mean a 15 per cent lower risk of breast cancer among all women and 19 per cent lower risk among premenopausal women.

Ferrari *et al.* (2013) focused on a different dietary component in their analysis of the EPIC (European Prospective Investigation into Cancer and Nutrition) study data. They investigated the relation between dietary fibre, its main food sources and breast cancer risk. The data showed that higher intake of fibre lowers the risk of breast cancer and the association was particularly strong with fibre from vegetables. This risk reduction was independent of the women's menopausal status or cancer hormone sensitivity. The UK Women's Cohort Study brought similar results – an increased fibre intake was linked to a lower breast cancer risk among British women (Cade *et al.*, 2007).

To assess the influence of a radical diet change and exercise on women at risk of breast cancer, Barnard *et al.* (2006) enlisted volunteers on a two week program. The women, who were all postmenopausal and overweight, agreed to follow a very low-fat, high-fibre diet consisting mainly of fruits, vegetables and wholegrains with very limited amounts of animal protein and daily aerobic exercise. At the end of the two-week period, their hormone levels decreased, including IGF-1 which dropped by as much as 19 per cent. The women also lost weight which is an important factor in breast cancer prevention and their blood sugar control improved. The serum isolated from the participants' blood samples before and at the end

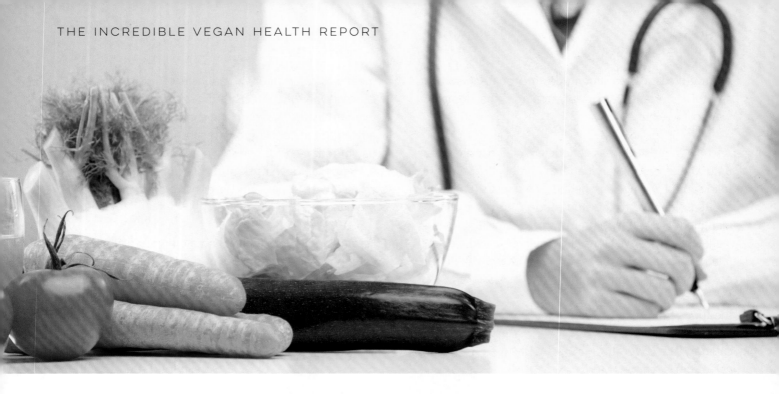

of the trial was used on breast cancer cells in a cell culture to see if there would be any difference in the cell growth. The results were of major importance as the after the intervention, the cancer cell growth was significantly slowed down and considerably more cancer cells died compared to pre-intervention.

Probably the best known case study of diet change and breast cancer is Professor Jane Plant who had conducted extensive research on diet and breast cancer to treat her own condition. What she found out and the hundreds of studies she based her decisions on led her to a conclusion that a vegan diet is necessary for successful breast cancer treatment (Plant, 2007). Her advice has since helped thousands of women and has been supported by many experts.

OVARIAN CANCER

The World Cancer Research Fund's 2007 report pointed out that ovarian cancer is most frequent in high income countries and also that there seems to be a direct relationship between vegetable intake and ovarian cancer – several studies showed that the higher the intake of vegetables, the lower the risk of this type of cancer.

In a large study of ovarian cancer patients and a healthy control group, it emerged that higher vegetable intake, particularly cruciferous vegetables, is linked to a lower risk of the disease, whilst dietary cholesterol and egg consumption was increasing the risk (Pan et al., 2004). A later analysis of studies focused on diet and ovarian cancer confirmed that indeed there's a strong association between cruciferous vegetables and a reduced cancer risk (Hu et al., 2015).

Dolecek et al. (2010) analysed pre-diagnosis diets of women with ovarian cancer and assessed how they're linked to survival and recovery. They found a strong link between high fruit and vegetable intake (particularly cruciferous vegetables) and higher chance of survival and the same applied to grains. On the other hand, higher intake of red meat, processed meat products and dairy was linked to a significantly lower chance of survival.

CERVIX CANCER

Various studies tried to assess whether a healthy diet can have a protective effect on the cervix, especially as the risk of cervix cancer is linked to HPV (human papilloma virus). And because most of these studies show a correlation between fruit and vegetable intake and an increased protection against cancerous lesions (García-Closas et al., 2005; Ghosh et al., 2008), a recent study was designed to look at overall dietary patterns and their effect on cervix health (Piyathilake et al., 2012). It revealed that women with unhealthy diets based on meat, fatty and processed foods have 3.3 times higher cervical cancer risk than women whose diets are plant-based and low in fat. Therefore, a low-fat plant-based diet can significantly reduce the risk of cervical cancer regardless of HPV infection.

PROSTATE CANCER

Berkow et al. (2007) reviewed studies on how diet influences the risk of prostate cancer and recovery in men who already have it. This led them to a conclusion that a diet high in saturated fat increases the risk of prostate cancer progression and death about three-fold compared to a diet low in saturated fat. The review also states that men who changed their diet to a plant-based one after diagnosis had a higher chance of recovery and so did men consuming soya, flaxseed and vegetables and fruit containing lycopene (a red pigment in fruit and vegetables – eg tomatoes, carrots, watermelon, papaya but also brown beans and asparagus). The authors suggest a plant-based diet high in fibre and phytonutrients for both prevention and as a part of prostate cancer treatment.

In an intervention, one-year long intervention study of men with low-risk prostate cancer that didn't require immediate treatment, half of the study group was assigned to a low-fat wholesome vegan diet (including at least one portion of soya foods a day) accompanied by moderate exercise and stress management techniques, and the other half served as a control group (Ornish et al., 2005). The men were monitored throughout and their blood analysed for changes in PSA (prostate cancer indicator). Six participants from the control group had to withdraw and undergo a conventional treatment but none of the intervention group did. PSA decreased by four per cent in the experimental group but increased by six per cent in the control group. The effect of participants' blood serum on cancer cells in vitro at the end of the study (after 12 months) was remarkable – serum from experimental group patients inhibited cancer cell growth by 70 per cent, whereas serum from control group patients inhibited growth by only 9 per cent.

Dr Ornish and his team later performed a unique study for which they enrolled 30 men with prostate cancer who did not undergo surgery or radiation therapy to treat their low-risk tumors (Ornish et al., 2008). These men agreed to undergo comprehensive lifestyle changes (low-fat, whole-foods, plant-based nutrition, stress management techniques, moderate exercise and participation in a psychosocial support group) and donated prostate needle biopsies at the beginning of the study and after three months of the lifestyle intervention. The study authors performed tests to compare gene expression and their up- or down-regulation in the prostate tissue. These tests detected (at the end of the intervention) down-regulation of many genes that significantly influence biological processes linked to cancer growth. Pathways involved in protein metabolism and modification, intracellular protein traffic and protein phosphorylation were significantly down-regulated, including the IGF-1 pathway.

A part of the European Prospective Investigation into Cancer and Nutrition (EPIC) study focused specifically on diet and prostate cancer (Allen et al., 2008). The scientific team examined consumption of animal foods, protein and calcium in relation to risk of prostate cancer among over 140,000 men. They found out that high intake of dairy protein was associated with an increased risk of prostate cancer and so was high calcium intake from dairy products (but not from non-dairy sources).

Another long-term study followed close to 9,000 men for prostate cancer diagnosis and mortality over at least two decades (Torfadottir et al., 2012). The results showed that milk intake, especially in the first 20 years of life, was associated with an increased risk of prostate cancer. Daily milk consumption in adolescence was associated with a 3.2-fold risk of advanced prostate cancer later in life.

Cow's milk naturally contains IGF-1 and stimulates the body to increase its own production of IGF-1 which can directly promote cancer growth. Both studies above raised concerns that this might be why dairy product consumption increases the risk of prostate cancer. High intake of animal fat has also been associated with increased testosterone levels and high testosterone levels may increase prostate cancer risk. An earlier study using data from 42 countries also showed a significant correlation between dairy products, cheese in particular, and prostate cancer (Ganmaa et al., 2002). After milk and dairy products, meat was linked to an increased risk of this cancer as well – both dairy products and meat contribute to elevated IGF-1 levels and contain considerable amounts of fat.

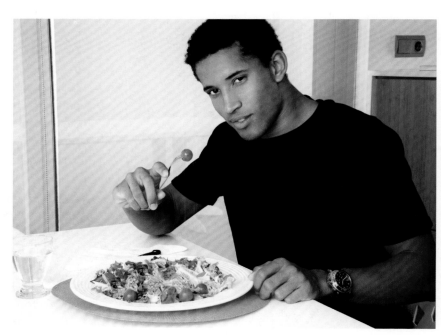

DIGESTIVE TRACT CANCERS

Many studies show that plant-based dietary patterns are linked to lower cancer rates and lower gastrointestinal cancer risk in particular (Tantamango-Bartley et al., 2013).

ORAL AND PHARYNGEAL CANCER

Oral and pharyngeal cancer is associated with lifestyle habits and apart from smoking and alcohol use, diet can play a considerable role in the prevention of this disease.

A large, long-term, multi-centre study of people from Italy and Switzerland investigated how the participants' diet impacts on both oral and pharyngeal cancer risk (Bravi et al., 2013). The results showed that higher consumption of fruit and vegetables was linked to a decreased risk of these two types of cancer, while milk and dairy products, eggs, red meat, potatoes and desserts increased the risk. With regard to nutrients, lower risk of cancer was associated with higher intake of vegetable protein, vegetable fat, polyunsaturated fatty acids and several vitamins and phytochemicals found in plant-based foods. On the other hand, nutrients contributing to a higher risk of oral and pharyngeal cancer were animal protein, animal fat, saturated fatty acids, cholesterol and retinol (vitamin A from animal sources). Combinations of low consumption of fruits and vegetables and high

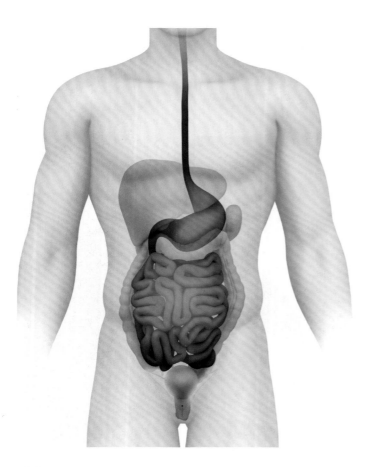

consumption of meat together with tobacco and alcohol led to 10-20-fold increased risk of oral and pharyngeal cancer.

Lucenteforte et al. (2009) reviewed data from nearly 50 studies on the relation between diet and the risk of oral and pharyngeal cancer. Fruit and vegetables and wholegrains were linked to a significantly decreased risk, leading the authors to recommend a diet high in these for cancer prevention.

A later review of case-control studies by Bravi et al. (2012a) came to a similar conclusion. They pointed out the findings that diets rich in fruit and vegetables can prevent oral and pharyngeal cancer are consistent across studies and that consumption of animal foods and alcohol markedly increases the risk.

ESOPHAGEAL CANCER

The same rules seem to apply to the prevention of esophageal cancer as to the above cancers. Li et al. (2013) analysed data from an enormous study of almost 500,000 people and reached the conclusion that the richer a diet is in fruit and vegetables, wholegrains and pulses, the lower the risk of esophageal cancer.

In another study of dietary patterns and cancer of the esophagus, Bravi et al. (2012b) discovered that diets high in meat, dairy, eggs and fatty foods increase the risk, whilst diets high in fruit and vegetables, pulses and fibre decrease the risk.

The latest exhaustive review on the subject agrees that a diet rich in fruits and vegetables and cessation of tobacco and alcohol use can significantly contribute to esophageal cancer prevention (Palladino-Davis et al., 2015).

GASTRIC CANCER

In 2009 Bertuccio et al. performed a study of 230 gastric cancer patients and compared their dietary patterns with 547 healthy people. They discovered a diet based on animal products and processed foods significantly increases cancer risk, while a diet high in fruit, vegetables and fibre-rich foods decreases it.

A meta-analysis and review of other studies on the same subject later conducted by Bertuccio et al. (2013) arrived at the conclusion that a wholesome diet including high consumption of fruits and vegetables may decrease the risk of gastric cancer by 25 percent, whilst a diet high in meat, high-fat dairy products, starchy foods and sweets can increase the risk by 50 per cent. And another scientific team performing an

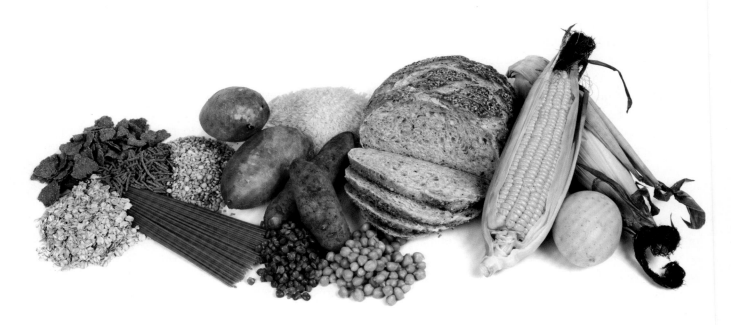

analysis of 23 studies confirmed this association with almost the same numbers (Shu *et al.*, 2013).

COLORECTAL CANCER

The preventative effect of a fibre-rich diet on colorectal cancer is now well-established. Dietary fibre increases stool bulk, promotes bowel movements, dilutes potential carcinogens in the gut and encourages health-beneficial bacteria. And because a vegan diet is naturally high in fibre and doesn't contain any animal protein and fat that encourage bacteria that produce toxic by-products, it has the biggest potential to protect against colorectal cancer.

Recently, The International Agency for Research on Cancer (IARC) evaluated the evidence to decide whether red and processed meat causes cancer (Bouvard *et al.*, 2015). The IARC's Working Group assessed more than 800 studies that investigated the association and, based on their conclusions, the World Health Organisation (WHO) announced that processed meat causes and red meat probably causes colorectal cancer. On top of that, processed meat was also strongly linked to stomach cancer. In this groundbreaking move and contrary to the meat industry's pressure, the WHO classified processed meat as carcinogenic and red meat as probably carcinogenic.

O'Keefe *et al.* (2015) performed a very interesting experiment. Based on the fact that rates of colon cancer are much higher in African Americans than in rural South Africans, they decided to swap their diets for two weeks and observe the results. Higher colon cancer rates are associated with higher animal protein and fat intake

and low fibre consumption, which is typical of an American diet. A rural African diet, on the other hand, is high in fibre and carbohydrates and low in fat.

On initial examination, African Americans had more polyps and growths in the colon. These differences were associated with profound differences in the intestinal bacteria. Africans had a high proportion of fibre fermenting bacteria which produce substances like butyrate that are anti-inflammatory and anti-cancerous. Americans had more bacteria that thrive on fats and metabolise bile acids, the products of which are carcinogenic.

The results of the diet swap were remarkable – it decreased the colon lining growth rate (proliferative rate which increases cancer risk) of the Americans to levels even lower than those of Africans at baseline, meanwhile the Africans' rate increased to levels greater than those of Americans at the start. At the same time, the markers of inflammation of Africans after two weeks of a high-fat, meat-based diet rose steeply and the inflammation markers of Americans on a low-fat, mostly plant-based diet decreased. Another significant result was that the gut bacteria of Americans on the high-fibre, low-fat diet diversified and the beneficial and protective species increased, whilst the American diet had the opposite effect on Africans, encouraging the growth of bacteria producing carcinogenic by-products.

Another arm of the comprehensive EPIC study focused on diet and colorectal cancer in a population of over 470,000 people from across Europe (Murphy *et al.*, 2012). Higher intake of fibre was linked to a significantly lower risk of colorectal cancer – for each ten grams of fibre a day, the risk of cancer decreased by 13 per cent. The study also revealed that the association was strongest for fibre from fruit, vegetables and grains and that people with high fibre diets also ate less meat in general.

And a meta-analysis of studies on the same topic agrees (Aune at al., 2011). A diet high in fibre, essentially a plant-based diet rich in fruit and vegetables, wholegrains and pulses, significantly decreases the risk of colorectal cancer. For each ten grams of fibre a day, the risk decreased by ten per cent.

An extensive analysis of studies that looked at pulse consumption (beans, lentils, soya, chickpeas, peas) and the risk of colorectal cancer also showed encouraging results (Zhu et al., 2015). People who ate more pulses had a lower risk of this type of cancer. In particular, both the intake of fibre from pulses and the intake of soya were associated with a lower colorectal cancer risk. Pulses are extremely nutritious, providing protein, fibre, vitamin E, vitamin B, selenium and lignans (plant chemical compounds) that have potential cancer-preventative effects. In addition, their protective properties were also attributed to compounds called flavonoids (only found in plant foods), which can inhibit the growth of tumour cells.

According to a study published in *PLoS Genetics*, a common genetic variant carried by one in three people significantly increases the risk of colorectal cancer for meat-eaters (Figueiredo et al., 2014). The study investigated how diet influences our genetic predisposition for cancer. It involved over 18,000 people from the US, Canada, Australia and Europe. It's generally agreed that meat consumption is associated with an increased risk of colorectal cancer but this study revealed that for about a third of the population who carry this specific genetic variant, the risk is even higher. On the other hand, the study also confirmed that vegetable, fruit and fibre intake lowers the risk.

PANCREATIC CANCER

Pancreatic cancer is also one of the cancers that have been directly linked to nutrition and dietary patterns. With traditional diets changing and being Westernised, some diseases are on the rise. The incidence of pancreatic cancer in China is increasing so Liu et al. (2014) conducted a study to investigate whether there is an association to dietary factors. They discovered that there was a strong link between meat consumption and pancreatic cancer and that fruit and vegetables and tea had protective effects.

A large study by Jansen et al. (2011) into the effects of diet on the risk of pancreatic cancer detected a significantly lower risk for people whose diets include citrus fruit, melons, berries, a variety of fruit in general, dark green vegetables, deep yellow vegetables, tomatoes, vegetables in general, beans and peas, wholegrains and other fibre-rich foods.

Bosetti et al. (2013) performed a very similar study in Italy and found very similar results as the studies above – a diet characterised by a high consumption of meat and other animal products, refined cereal products and sugars considerably increases the risk of pancreatic cancer risk, whereas a diet rich in fruit and vegetables is linked to a low risk.

And a Harvard study focused specifically on nut consumption in relation to pancreatic cancer revealed that people who eat a small portion of nuts at least two times a week have up to 35 per cent lower risk of this type of cancer (Bao et al., 2013). People eating nuts on a regular basis also happened to have higher intake of fruit and vegetables but the protective effect of nut intake remained even after the other dietary factors were accounted for.

LUNG CANCER

The results from the lung cancer section of the EPIC study examining the link between fruit and vegetable consumption and lung cancer showed that regular fruit and vegetable intake reduces the risk of lung cancer in both non-smokers and smokers (Büchner et al., 2010a). When the smokers' data were analysed further, the scientists found out that an increased variety in fruit and vegetable consumption decreases lung cancer risk further (Büchner et al., 2010b).

Hosseini et al. (2014) performed a study of 242 lung cancer patients and compared their health and lifestyle to a large control group of age and sex matched healthy people. In the analysis of their diets, they found out that fruit, vegetable and vegetable oil consumption was linked to lower risk of lung cancer, whilst diets containing red meat, liver, animal fats, cheese and refined cereals was associated with a higher risk.

And another remarkable review study shows that compounds found in cruciferous vegetables (eg Brussels sprouts, broccoli and kale) may protect against lung cancer (Lam et al., 2009). This review of 30 studies found that the risk for lung cancer was around 20 per cent lower in those who ate the most cruciferous vegetables compared to those consuming the least.

BLADDER CANCER

Several studies have linked diet to bladder cancer. Since the metabolic products of nutrients are excreted through the urinary tract, diet can play an important role here.

The EPIC study of almost 500,000 people from across Europe examined dietary intake of main nutrients and their impact on the risk of bladder cancer (Allen et al., 2013). One nutrient seemed to be of crucial importance – protein – but not all protein is the same. According to the results, the higher the intake of animal protein, the higher the risk of bladder cancer – just a three per cent increase in the consumption of animal protein was associated with a 15 per cent higher risk of bladder cancer. On the other hand, plant protein intake lowered the risk – a two per cent increase in plant protein intake was associated with a 23 per cent lower risk of bladder cancer.

It has been suggested that the high nitrosamine content of some processed meat products may increase the risk, that the difference in amino acid profiles of animal and plant protein plays a role too and last but not least, animal protein increases the levels of IGF-1 in the body – one of the main cancer promoters.

Ferrucci et al. (2010) investigated meat-related compounds including nitrate, nitrite, heterocyclic amines (HCAs) and polycyclic aromatic hydrocarbons (PAHs) and their links to bladder cancer. Nitrate and nitrite are compounds added to processed meat for preservation and enhance colour and flavour. Both nitrate and nitrite are metabolised into N-nitroso compounds (NOCs) which can cause cancer. The source of nitrate is crucial because nitrate from plants behaves differently and does not produce carcinogenic compounds. Other important risk factors are heterocyclic amines (HCAs) and polycyclic aromatic hydrocarbons (PAHs) formed in meats prepared by high temperature cooking methods. These compounds are known carcinogens. In the Ferrucci et al. study, there was a link between high consumption of red meat, nitrite and the combination of nitrite and nitrate from processed meat and bladder cancer. The authors also observed an association between HCA intake and cancer risk.

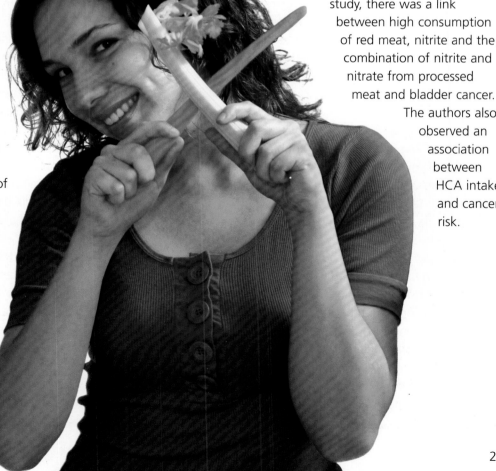

A WORD ON SOYA

Many people are unsure about soya and cancer because of phytoestrogens (plant hormones) naturally occurring in soya-based foods. The type of phytoestrogens present in soya are called isoflavones. Isoflavones are plant substances (most commonly found in soya foods but also in other pulses such as beans and lentils), which can act as very mild oestrogens in the body. However, the oestrogen effects of isoflavones are much less powerful than those of oestrogens – about 1,000-10,000 times weaker. Isoflavones bind to the same receptors in the body as oestrogens and this is why isoflavones have a balancing effect when the levels of oestrogens are low, such as during the menopause, and can ease menopause symptoms. Isoflavones can also reduce the effect of oestrogens when the hormone levels are high, and then essentially reduce the risk of oestrogen sensitive cancers.

SOYA AND BREAST CANCER
To establish whether soya is safe for women with breast cancer, almost 10,000 women were followed for several years and their diets analysed. To examine the possibility of cultural and lifestyle influences, the study included North American and Chinese women. The results of this largest study to date on soya and breast cancer showed that for all women alike, soya consumption after the breast cancer diagnosis slightly decreased the risk of death and significantly decreased the risk of breast cancer recurrence (Nechuta et al., 2012).

The Shanghai Breast Cancer Survival Study looked at over 5,000 women diagnosed with breast cancer an average of four years previously and their diets. Results showed that those who ate more soya foods (around 11 grams of soya protein a day, the amount in around one and a half servings of soya foods like tofu or soya milk) were 29 per cent less likely to die from the disease and had a 32 per cent lower risk of recurrence. The researchers concluded that for women with breast cancer, consuming soya foods improves prognosis (Shu et al., 2009).

The results of the two studies above are in agreement with yet another recent study. Zhang et al. (2012) found out that breast cancer patients who ate on average 17.3 mg soya isoflavones a day (equivalent to a small tofu portion, a glass of soya milk, soya sausage or a small slice of tempeh) had up to 38 per cent lower risk of death and higher soya intake was also linked to a significantly lower risk of cancer recurrence.

And not only is soya consumption safe for women at risk or with breast cancer, it can also help prevent it. According to a study of more than 1,500 Asian American women, eating soya foods during childhood can reduce the risk of breast cancer by up to 60 per cent (Korde et al., 2009). In this study, the greatest protective effect was seen in those eating soya at least six times a month, compared to less than three, from childhood onwards. A further protective effect was also seen in those who ate soya during adolescence and adulthood. Previous studies have shown similar protective effects of eating soya in adolescence, such as Shu et al. (2001) who observed that women who ate the most soya had up to 50 per cent lower risk of breast cancer later in life.

SOYA AND ENDOMETRIAL CANCER
The results of a long-term (over 13 years) study of nearly 50,000 women of all ethnicities revealed that regular intake of isoflavones can significantly reduce the risk of endometrial cancer (Ollberding et al., 2012). Endometrial cancer usually means cancer of the inner lining of the uterus but it can spread or affect surrounding tissues and is hormone sensitive. The hormone normalising effect of isoflavones has been linked to the reduced risk of this type of cancer and the amount that's been shown to reduce the risk equals roughly one glass of soya milk or one serving of soya-based food a day.

SOYA AND PROSTATE CANCER
Yan and Spitznagel (2009) conducted a meta-analysis of studies on soya and prostate cancer. The results of this analysis suggest that consumption of soya foods is associated with a reduced risk of prostate cancer. Non-fermented soya foods (tofu, soya milk, etc.) seemed to have stronger preventative effects.

CARDIOVASCULAR DISEASE

Cardiovascular disease (CVD) is a general term for diseases of the heart or blood vessels. The main types of CVD are coronary heart disease, stroke and peripheral arterial disease.

Coronary heart disease (CHD) occurs when the flow of blood into the heart is limited or blocked by a build-up of plaques in the coronary arteries (two major blood vessels supplying the heart with oxygen-rich blood). Restricted blood supply to the heart can cause angina (chest pain) and if the supply is completely blocked it causes collapse of the heart muscle – a heart attack.

A stroke is a condition that occurs when the blood supply to a part of the brain is severely limited or blocked. If the brain cannot get enough oxygen through blood supply, it can cause brain damage very quickly and may result in death.

Peripheral arterial disease (or peripheral vascular disease) occurs when there's a blockage in the arteries supplying blood to the limbs, usually the legs. The most common symptom is leg pain when walking or exercising the legs.

All these blockages occur as a result of atherosclerosis – a condition where arteries become narrower because of fatty build-ups known as plaques or atheroma. Plaque is made of cholesterol, fatty substances, cellular waste products (as white blood cells attach themselves to the cholesterol deposits in an attempt to dissolve them), calcium and fibrin (a clotting material in the blood).

The plaques cause affected arteries to harden and narrow, thus restricting blood flow. If a plaque tears away or ruptures or if an artery becomes too narrow to function properly, it can block the blood supply to vital organs and cause any of the above conditions.

There are many risk factors for CVD, including high blood pressure (hypertension), smoking, high blood

cholesterol levels, diabetes, physical inactivity, being overweight or obese and a family history of heart disease. However, most of these are modifiable and a substantial change can be achieved through diet.

PREVENTION

When the extensive EPIC study analysed data on CVD from the British population to examine whether vegetarians have a lower risk of the disease than omnivores, it brought predictable results (Crowe et al., 2013). Vegetarians had on average much healthier weight, cholesterol levels and blood pressure – all crucial risk factors for CVD – and as a result, their risk of CVD was 32 per cent lower than in the omnivore population.

In terms of blood cholesterol, vegans had the lowest levels compared to vegetarians and meat-eaters (Bradbury et al., 2014). This could be to a small degree attributed to weight differences but diet composition is by far the biggest factor.

A previous EPIC analysis looking only at the blood pressure of British participants showed that vegans have the lowest and meat-eaters the highest blood pressure; vegetarians and pescatarians were in the middle (Appleby et al., 2002). Accordingly, vegans had the lowest risk of suffering from hypertension. The same conclusion was reached in the Adventist Health Study 2 that was following American and Canadian subjects (Pettersen et al., 2012). In this study, vegans had 63 per cent lower risk of hypertension than meat eating participants.

Huang et al. (2012) analysed seven studies with a total of 124,706 participants. They found that vegetarians have a significantly lower CVD mortality – their risk was 29 per cent lower than in omnivores.

And when analysing data from studies on diet and stroke, He et al. (2006) observed that the higher the intake of fruit and vegetables, the lower the risk of stroke. People who consumed more than five portions a day had a 26 per cent lower risk of stroke.

To test whether a low-fat wholesome vegan diet can achieve measurable differences in CVD risk factors over a period as short as one week, McDougall *et al.* (2014) assigned volunteers on a residential program where they were tested before and after and all their meals were prepared by professionals. The participants were not limited in their food intake. After one week on this vegan diet, they achieved weight loss, decrease in cholesterol levels and blood pressure, and better blood sugar control. In conclusion, just seven days of this lifestyle achieved substantial favourable changes in common risk factors for CVD and metabolic diseases.

TREATMENT

Intensive lifestyle changes have been shown to be able to achieve significant improvements in people who have CVD or are at risk.

Dr Ornish was among the first experts who started advocating a vegan diet for the treatment of CVD. He and his team performed a long-term study that involved diet and lifestyle changes and followed the participants for five years (Ornish *et al.*, 1998). Patients with moderate to severe CVD were assigned to an intensive lifestyle change group or to a no-change control group. The lifestyle change group were asked to consume a low-fat almost vegan diet, do moderate aerobic exercise, practice stress management and stop smoking. Throughout and at the end of the study (after five years) the vegan group had a significant improvement in blood vessel health – the plaques in the arteries were markedly reduced and the blood flow improved – whilst in the control group, the narrowing of the arteries (atherosclerosis) steadily increased.

Patients in the experimental group lost excess weight, their LDL ('bad') cholesterol levels decreased by 40 per cent after just one year and remained 20 per cent below baseline at five years. None of the experimental group patients took lipid-lowering drugs during the study. The vegan patients also had a 91 per cent reduction in reported frequency of angina after one year and a 72 per cent reduction after five years.

Dod *et al.* (2010) enrolled people with or at risk of CVD on a three-month program that required them to change their diet to a low-fat vegan one, do three hours of moderate exercise a week and practice stress management. At the end of the study, the participants' blood vessel function and blood flow had significantly improved, their cholesterol levels were reduced and their inflammatory markers significantly decreased.

In an intervention study of 198 people with CVD, 177 adhered to the diet principles (followed on average for 3.7 years) which were for wholegrains, pulses (lentils, beans, soya, peas, chickpeas), vegetables and fruit to form the basis of the diet (Esselstyn *et al.*, 2014). Participants were also encouraged to take a multivitamin and vitamin B12 supplement and advised to use of flaxseed meal as an additional source of omega-6 and omega-3 essential fatty acids. Apart from animal-based foods, patients were also told to avoid added oils and processed foods that contain oils, avocado, nuts, sugary foods and drinks and excess salt. In the group of adherent patients, 112 reported angina at the beginning and 104 of them experienced improvement or resolution of symptoms during the follow-up period. Among adherent patients with

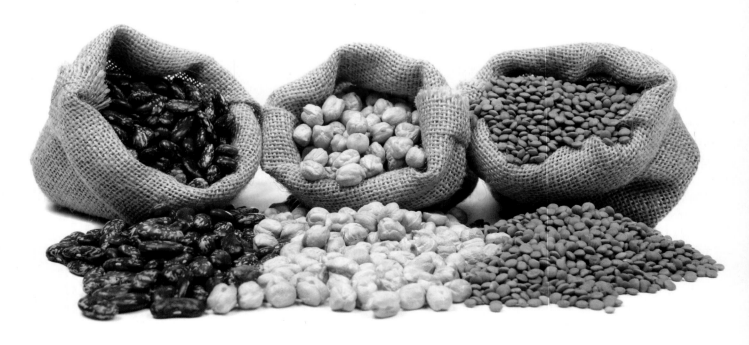

severely affected (blocked) coronary arteries, results showed disease reversal in 39 cases and 27 participants were able to avoid surgery that was previously recommended. Only one cardiac event related to the progression of CVD occurred in the group of adherent patients – a non-fatal stroke. On the other hand, 13 of the 21 (62 per cent) non-adherent participants experienced adverse events. These included two sudden cardiac deaths, one heart transplant, two strokes, four surgeries with stent placement, three coronary artery bypass surgeries and one carotid artery surgery.

The above is just one of Dr Esselstyn's studies but his purely plant-based approach to preventing and reversing CVD is internationally renowned. He has countless case studies proving the effectiveness of low-fat vegan diets (Esselstyn, 2007).

A team of scientists from Harvard studied how diet impacts on heart attack survivors. Those who changed their diet and increased their fibre intake (moving towards a plant-based diet) post heart attack had significantly higher chances of survival (Li et al., 2014a). In particular, greater intake of fibre from wholegrains was found to be very beneficial. Increasing fibre consumption was also strongly associated with lower mortality from all causes, as well as cardiovascular disease.

On the other hand, patients who followed a low carbohydrate diet high in animal sources of protein and fat had a higher all-cause and cardiovascular mortality (Li et al., 2014b). The study authors did not find any health benefits from adherence to a low carbohydrate diet.

A review of studies on how diets generally recommended for people with/at risk of CVD or diabetes or wholesome vegan diets affect human health arrived at a conclusion that vegan diets are clearly better for both, improving cardiovascular health and blood sugar control (Trepanowski and Varady, 2015).

CATARACTS

A cataract is a clouding of the lens in the eye, either formed of proteins or pigments, that develops slowly and leads to a decrease in vision. It can eventually lead to blindness.

The Oxford part of the enormous EPIC study included over 27,000 people and one of the studied health aspects in this population sample was the relationship between diet and cataracts (Appleby et al., 2011). This study showed a strong relation between cataract risk

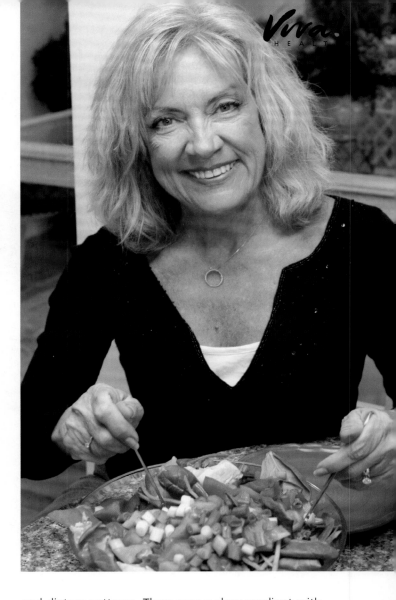

and dietary patterns. There was a clear gradient with the risk of cataracts being highest in high meat-eaters and decreasing progressively in low meat-eaters, pescaterians, vegetarians and vegans. Vegans had the lowest possible risk of cataracts, 40 per cent lower than meat-eaters. In a further analysis, high intake of cholesterol, saturated fats and protein was significantly linked to cataracts.

Pastor-Valero (2013) studied the prevalence of cataracts in a Spanish population. She discovered a direct relationship – with increasing intake of fruit and vegetables, the risk of cataracts decreased. The conclusion of her study was that high intakes of fruit and vegetables as well as vitamins C and E (the sources of which are plant-based foods) are associated with a significantly lower risk of cataracts.

And when Rautiainen et al. (2014) studied the risk of cataracts in a Swedish population, they observed the same patterns as the studies above – the more antioxidant-rich foods in the diet, the lower the risk of cataracts. The major contributors to antioxidant intake were fruit and vegetables, wholegrains and coffee.

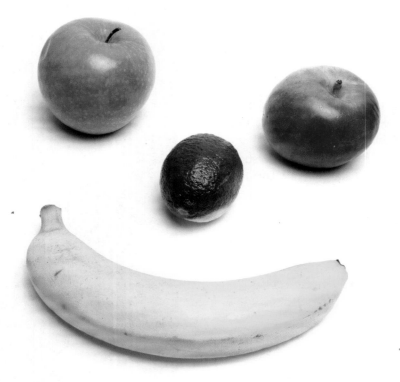

CHRONIC OBSTRUCTIVE PULMONARY DISEASE (COPD)

Chronic obstructive pulmonary disease (COPD) is the generic name for a cluster of lung diseases including chronic bronchitis, emphysema and chronic obstructive airways disease. People with COPD have difficulties breathing, primarily due to the narrowing of their airways and the condition progressively worsens over time. Chronic bronchitis is inflammation of the air passages with airflow obstruction and causes a long-term cough with mucus. Emphysema is a condition causing destruction of the lung tissue.

Varraso et al. (2015) analysed data from a large study of over 120,000 people in order to study the effect of diet on the risk of COPD. There was a significant negative association between the risk of COPD and a healthy diet. People eating the healthiest diet (based on wholegrains, fruit and vegetables, nuts and seeds, pulses and low in red and processed meats, refined grains and sugary drinks) had 33 per cent lower risk of developing COPD.

When the association between diet and COPD was studied in a UK population, diets rich in fruit, vegetables, polyunsaturated fats and wholegrains were shown to convey protection against impaired lung function and COPD (Shaheen et al., 2010).

Similar results were found when COPD and lung function were studied in relation to fibre intake (Kan et al., 2008). The researchers found that lung function is significantly better in people with the highest intake of fibre in general (from all plant sources combined) and particularly with cereal and fruit fibre. The higher the intake of these foods, the lower the risk of COPD. The authors suggested the protective effect of fibre on lung health is probably due to the anti-inflammatory and antioxidant properties of fibre.

A plant-based diet can also help manage the condition in people who suffer from COPD and reduce the risk of premature death. Almost 3,000 men from across Europe with COPD were followed for 20 years and at the end of the study all the data were analysed (Walda et al., 2002). High fruit and vitamin E intake significantly reduced mortality risk. More specifically, a 100 g increase in daily fruit intake was associated with a 24 per cent lower COPD mortality risk. For vitamin E, a 5 mg increase in daily intake reduced the risk by 23 per cent. A vegan diet is naturally rich in vitamin E as all main food sources of this vitamin are of plant origin.

These results are supported by an earlier study of diet and lung function of British men (Butland et al., 2000). The researchers measured middle-aged men's lung function and analysed their diets over the period of five years. Good lung function was linked to high intakes of vitamin C, vitamin E, ß-carotene, citrus fruits, apples and fruit juice.

All the studies above and more show that plant-based foods rich in antioxidants and fibre have a beneficial effect on lung health and can prevent COPD.

DIABETES

Diabetes is a condition caused by the pancreas failing to produce the hormone insulin or producing insufficient quantities. Another cause is insulin resistance – the body cells' inability to react to insulin. Insulin is a hormone produced by the pancreas and acts as a key, allowing glucose into the body's cells. Glucose is a vital source of energy for cells and is the main fuel for the brain and body's processes. In diabetics, blood sugar levels rise too high and this can damage blood vessels and cause nerve damage but it also has a negative effect on health overall, increasing cholesterol levels and the risk of heart disease.

TYPE 1 DIABETES

Type 1 diabetes is less common and typically develops early in life when the immune system attacks the insulin-producing cells in the pancreas and destroys them. It results in the body being unable to produce insulin and therefore use glucose. Type 1 diabetics have to inject insulin on a regular basis.

Evidence is increasing that a combination of susceptible genes and early exposure to cow's milk is responsible for this self-harming reaction of the body. It might be also triggered by a virus or other infection. Several gene variants have been identified as contributing to type 1 diabetes susceptibility but only a small proportion of genetically susceptible individuals – less than 10 per cent – go on to develop the disease (Knip et al., 2005). This implies that environmental factors are necessary to trigger the autoimmune reaction which destroys insulin producing cells.

If an individual has a certain combination of genes making them more susceptible to type 1 diabetes, the environmental trigger is the crucial factor in the disease development but if the trigger is avoided, diabetes may be avoided. The hypothesis that cow's milk is the main trigger was put forward in the 1990's (Karjalainen et al., 1992; Gerstein, 1994; kerblom and Knip, 1998) and has been progressively more accepted ever since. The theory is as follows (Campbell and Campbell, 2004; Knip et al., 2005):

A baby with a susceptible genetic make-up is exposed to cows' milk early in life, perhaps through an infant formula. The baby's immune system might be further compromised by a virus infection, increasing the risk for type 1 diabetes. When the milk proteins reach the small intestine they are not fully digested – ie broken down into individual amino acids – but are instead broken down into amino acid chains. These fragments may be absorbed through the gut wall into the blood where the immune system recognises them as foreign intruders and begins attacking them through an immune response. Coincidentally, the structure of some of these fragments is identical to the surface structure of insulin producing cells (ß-cells) in the pancreas (Karjalainen et al., 1992; Martin et al., 1991) and the body cannot distinguish between the two. Pancreas ß-cells are therefore attacked and eventually destroyed by the immune system as well as the milk protein fragments and the infant becomes diabetic. Type 1 diabetes is irreversible as the cells cannot regenerate.

The process of ß-cell destruction can be fast and aggressive, leading to disease manifestation within a few months, or it can be slow and last for years, in some cases even more than 10 years with ß-cells being gradually destroyed over this period with each exposure (Knip et al., 2005). The fast progression of the disease is rare (Knip, 2002).

Research has established which milk proteins are responsible for this dramatic autoimmune reaction. Karjalainen et al. (1992) suggest that the main one is bovine serum albumin (BSA), which is different in structure to human albumin (milk protein). They tested the blood of type 1 diabetic and non-diabetic children for the presence of antibodies against incompletely digested BSA. The results were astonishing – all diabetic children had antibody levels as much as seven times higher than the healthy children and there was no overlap in the antibody levels between the diabetic and healthy children – ie all diabetic children had high levels but none of the non-diabetic children did.

After that, a number of studies ensued and all but one found markedly elevated levels of BSA antibodies in the blood of diabetic children (Hammond-McKibben and Dosch, 1997).

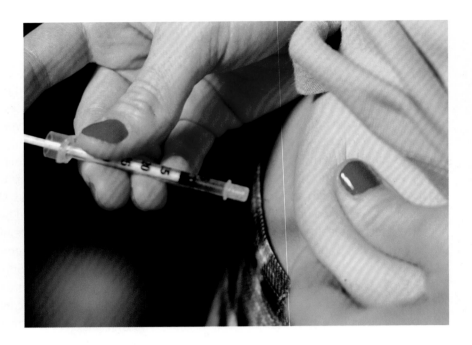

Another protein abundant in cow's milk is ß-casein, which also generates a specific immune response (Cavallo *et al.*, 1996). The structure of human ß-casein is similar in many respects to bovine ß-casein (from cow's milk) but 30 per cent of the molecule is different in structure. This difference is assumed to be the reason why the immune system reacts to it. Again there are structural similarities between bovine ß-casein and the surface molecules of ß-cells in the pancreas, just as there is with BSA, provoking an immunological cross-reactivity – the immune system attacks ß-casein molecules as well as the ß-cells.

A Chilean study conducted around the same time focused on the combination of susceptible genes and cow's milk (Perez-Bravo *et al.*, 1996). The findings revealed that genetically susceptible children weaned too early onto cow's milk-based formula had 13 times greater risk of developing type 1 diabetes than children breast-fed for at least three months and who did not have susceptible genes.

In 2000, an extensive study of children from 40 different countries confirmed a link between diet and type 1 diabetes (Muntoni *et al.*, 2000). The study set out to examine the relationship between dietary energy from major food groups and type 1 diabetes. Energy intake per se was not associated with type 1 diabetes but energy from animal sources (meat and dairy foods) showed a significant association whereas energy from plant sources was inversely associated with diabetes. In other words, the more meat and milk in the diet, the higher the incidence of diabetes and the more plant-based foods in the diet, the lower the incidence.

In the meantime, it was discovered that there are five autoantibodies – antibodies which will attack their own host body – and the presence of these autoantibodies can predict the development of type 1 diabetes (Knip, 2002). In addition to the two which attack ß-cells, together with two supporting antibodies, there is one which will attack insulin itself. It was suggested that cow's insulin present in formula milk increases the formation of these insulin antibodies (Vaarala *et al.*, 1999). A Finnish study of children at increased risk of

type 1 diabetes (having at least one close relative with the disease) showed that the immune system of infants given cow's milk formula as early as three-months old, reacted strongly to cow's insulin by forming these specific antibodies (Paronen *et al.*, 2000).

Results of another study following infants from birth (kerblom *et al.*, 2002) showed that exclusively breastfeeding for only a short period followed by the introduction of cow's milk, predisposed these children to ß-cell-destroying autoimmune reactions by inducing formation of four culprit autoantibodies. Other population studies have shown that if three or four of these antibodies are present in blood, the risk of developing type 1 diabetes in the next five to 10 years is 60-100 per cent (Knip *et al.*, 2005).

A recent study showed that introducing cow's milk into the diet of infants between six and 12 months of age increased four-fold the likelihood of developing type 1 diabetes later in childhood (Villagrán-García *et al.*, 2015). And another study examining the link between diabetes and cow's milk warned that early introduction of cow's milk is a risk factor for type 1 diabetes (Kamal Alanani and Alsulaimani, 2013).

There is enough evidence linking cow's milk consumption to type 1 diabetes that it's advisable not to consume it or feed it to children. If the autoimmune reaction is triggered, it's irreversible and type 1 diabetes has to be managed with insulin and possibly other drugs throughout life. A plant-based diet can provide all nutrients even for infants and children and can help prevent autoimmune reactions.

TYPE 2 DIABETES

In type 2 diabetes, the body can still make some insulin but not enough or it fails to react to insulin as it should (insulin resistance). Lifestyle and environmental factors play an enormous role in type 2 diabetes. Therefore, even individuals with susceptible genes, or people who have already developed type 2 diabetes, don't necessarily have to live with the condition for the rest of their lives.

Comparing diets and diabetes rates in different countries reveals that as carbohydrate intake goes down and fat intake goes up, the number of diabetics rapidly increases (Campbell & Campbell, 2004; Barnard, 2007). The difference cannot be ascribed to genetics as when people move to countries where the 'Western' style diet predominates and they adopt these eating habits, their rates of type 2 diabetes increase above the national average (Tsunehara et al., 1990).

Research suggests that eating just one serving of meat per week significantly increases the risk of diabetes. A study looked at the link between meat intake and the occurrence of diabetes in 8,000 adult Seventh Day Adventists, all of whom were non-diabetic at the start of the study (Vang et al., 2008). Those who followed a 'low-meat' diet over the 17 years of this long-term study had a staggering 74 per cent increase in their risk of developing type 2 diabetes compared to participants who followed a meat-free diet for the same period. Part of this difference was attributable to obesity and/or weight gain but even after allowances were made for this, meat intake remained an important risk factor.

A study published in 2004 produced an outstanding discovery (Petersen et al., 2004) and confirmed the findings of previous studies (Phillips et al., 1996; Krssak et al., 1999). The researchers tested young healthy

adults, whose family members were diabetic, for insulin resistance. Those who tested positive were found to have microscopic drops of fat in their muscle cells. This fat interfered with the cells' ability to correctly react to insulin. Even though their bodies produced sufficient insulin, fat inside their cells inhibited the correct reactions.

Muscle cells normally store small quantities of fat as an energy reserve but in the insulin-resistant people fat had built up to levels which were 80 per cent higher than in other young (healthy) people. Even though the affected people were slim, fat had nevertheless accumulated in their cells. The fat particles were intramyocellular lipids which start accumulating many years before type 2 diabetes manifests. It was then confirmed by other studies that insulin resistance in muscle and liver cells is strongly linked to fat storage in these tissues (Delarue and Magnan, 2007; Morino et al., 2006).

In order to understand the extent to which diet influences intracellular fat metabolism, another study was conducted (Sparks et al., 2005). Young healthy men were put on a special, high-fat diet that drew 50 per cent of its calories from fat – a diet not too different from that which many people in Western countries consume. After just three days, intracellular lipids had increased considerably, showing that accumulation of fat inside cells is fast and diet-dependant.

A study of cell metabolism in relation to insulin resistance revealed that elevated fat levels in blood and/or intramuscular fat accumulation can cause reduction in mitochondrial function which is crucial for insulin sensitivity (Hoeks, et al., 2010). Mitochondria are in every cell and they perform many metabolic functions, including taking part in sugar and fat metabolism.

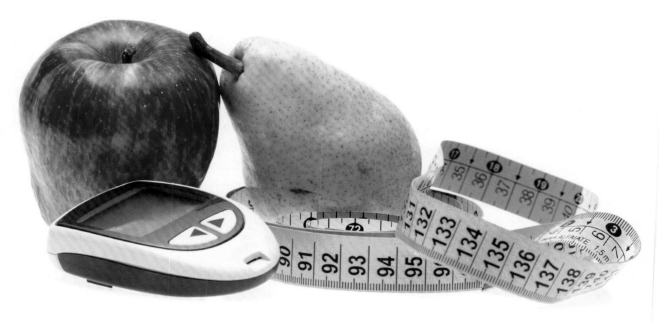

Based on the above, Gojda et al. (2013) studied insulin sensitivity, intramyocellular lipids and mitochondria in healthy vegans and omnivores without close relatives with diabetes. The study participants were matched for age, weight, height and waist circumference. The tests discovered that vegans had higher insulin sensitivity, less intromyocellular lipids and slightly more mitochondria. Their glucose metabolism was overall more efficient and sensitive than in the other group. Vegans also had significantly lower cholesterol levels and their blood lipid profile was much better than that of omnivores.

Research shows that with the right diet it is possible to decrease blood sugar, limit medication, cut the risk of complications and even reverse type 2 diabetes.

One of the first studies to test the effects of a plant-based, low-fat diet and exercise on a group of 40 type 2 diabetic patients, had outstanding results – 36 of the patients were able to discontinue all medication after only 26 days (Barnard et al., 1982). The same research group later demonstrated that the benefits of this diet are long-term and last for years, if the diet is adhered to (Barnard et al., 1983).

In one of the groundbreaking studies that followed, researchers employed a combination of diet change and exercise (Barnard et al., 1994). The subjects were 197 men with type 2 diabetes and after just three weeks of a low-fat plant-based diet, 140 of them were able to discontinue their medication.

A study with a different angle involved 21 diabetics with diabetic neuropathy (characterised by numbness and shooting or burning pains in the lower limbs), who volunteered to follow a vegan, whole food diet and exercise programme for 25 days (Crane and Sample, 1994). Within 16 days, 17 of the patients reported that the neuropathic pain had been completely alleviated. Although the numbness persisted, it was noticeably improved within the 25 days of the programme.

And a new study on the same subject agrees that a low-fat vegan diet can reduce diabetic neuropathy (Bunner et al., 2015). In this study, diabetics were either assigned to a low-fat vegan diet or to a control group with no diet change. Everyone was also given a vitamin B12 supplement for the 20 weeks of the study. At the end, the vegan group achieved improved blood-sugar control with some patients needing to have their medication reduced. They also experienced healthy weight-loss, a decrease in cholesterol levels and much greater reduction of pain compared to the control group.

A 2006 study, conducted by the Physicians Committee for Responsible Medicine with the George Washington University and the University of Toronto, tested the health benefits of a low-fat vegan diet emphasising foods with a low glycemic index value (low in fast-absorbing sugars) and excluding all animal products on people with type 2 diabetes. It was compared to a diet based on the American Diabetes Association (ADA) guidelines which restricted calorie intake and limited carbohydrates (Barnard et al., 2006). Portions of vegetables, grains, fruits and pulses were unlimited. Over the 22-week study, 43 per cent of the vegan group and 26 per cent of the ADA group reduced their diabetes medications. Furthermore, the vegan group lost an average of almost one stone (13 pounds), compared with just over half a stone (9 pounds) in the ADA group.

Overall quality of this vegan diet was compared to the ADA diet on the basis of the Alternate Healthy Eating Index (AHEI), which is used to estimate the risk of chronic diseases (Turner-McGrievy et al., 2008). It employs a scoring system which assesses several dietary behaviours and rates food and nutrient intakes. The vegan group improved in every AHEI food category (vegetables, fruit, nuts and soya protein, ratio of white to red meat, cereal fibre, trans fat, polyunsaturated to saturated fat ratio) and significantly improved the overall AHEI score. The ADA group improved in only two categories (nuts and soya protein, polyunsaturated to saturated fat ratio) and did not improve the overall AHEI score of the group. An increase in AHEI score was also associated with decreases in HbA1c value (which measures blood sugar levels over time) and weight.

Following the success of the previous studies, a 74-week clinical trial using a low-fat vegan diet was conducted (Barnard et al., 2009a). Participants were

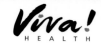

type 2 diabetics and they were randomly assigned to a low-fat vegan diet or a diet following ADA guidelines. HbA1c changes (measure of blood sugar control) from the beginning of the study to 74 weeks, or to the last available value before any medication adjustment, were -0.40 points for the vegan group and 0.01points for the conventional diet group. In patients whose medication did not need to be adjusted, HbA1c fell 1.23 points over the initial 22 weeks, compared to 0.38 points in the ADA group. Glycemic control, therefore, improved significantly more in the vegan group.

The reduction in triglycerides (fats in blood) in the vegan group was also remarkable as was the decrease in cholesterol levels (20.4mg/dl in contrast to just 6.8mg/dl in the conventional group). Both groups managed to lose weight but unlike the vegan participants, volunteers on the conventional (ADA) diet had restricted calorie intake whilst the vegan group did not.

A similar study was conducted in Europe, where half of the study participants (all type 2 diabetics) were assigned to a plant-based diet for 24 weeks and the other half served as a control group (Kahleova et al., 2011). The plant-based diet was based on fruit and vegetables, wholegrains, pulses, nuts and seeds. Both groups received a vitamin B12 supplement and were encouraged to do gentle exercise in the second half of the study. At the end, 43 per cent of participants in the experimental group but only five per cent in the control group had to have their medication reduced. An increase in insulin sensitivity was significantly greater in the experimental group than in the control group and the experimental group also lost much more fat. This was accompanied by a reduction in oxidative stress markers in the group following a plant-based diet which indicates better health.

Volunteers participating in some of the above studies preferred the vegan diet not only because it was effective but also because they found it better than the diet previously recommended. Participants in the 74-week study were repeatedly asked to rate the acceptability of their diets (Barnard et al., 2009b) and the results showed that patients initially felt more restricted by the ADA diet and at the end of the study reported that the vegan diet was as acceptable as the conventional diet. These findings suggest that following a diet that reverses diabetes is no harder than following a conventionally recommended diet which produces only minor changes in metabolism.

Parallel to these intervention studies, another research

CASE STUDY: PETER SCOTT, LANCASHIRE

After being diagnosed, I became a typical example – fat around the middle, high BMI, high cholesterol and high blood sugar. I had no energy, would cough a lot despite not smoking and didn't sleep well. But then I heard about the vegan diet. After just four weeks on the diet, my blood pressure started to fall towards normal levels. All my blood readings were approaching or within normal ranges. After eight weeks on a vegan diet, I lost 1.7 stone. Four months later, I'm no longer obese and my blood results show I'm no longer diabetic. I feel fitter, I sleep well, I wake up more quickly even without coffee and I've stopped the coughing probably because I stopped drinking milk. I continue to enjoy the diet and my new way of life. Thank you again, Viva!, for your work and your help.

group focused on analysing dietary patterns of 2,875 volunteers without diabetes and determined their risk of diabetes by repeated measurements of basic indicators – blood glucose, insulin concentrations, cholesterol levels, and waist circumference (Liu et al., 2009). Their findings were clear: consumption of a diet based mainly on plant foods protects against insulin resistance, while refined grains, high-fat dairy, desserts and sweets and sugary soft drinks promote insulin resistance.

Vegetarians have lower rates of diabetes than the general population but one study looked at the vegetarian dietary patterns across North America more closely to identify any differences (Tonstad et al., 2009). The authors discovered that vegans had the lowest prevalence of type 2 diabetes, only 2.9 per cent, lacto-ovo vegetarians 3.2 per cent, pesco-vegetarians 4.8 per cent, semi-vegetarians 6.1 per cent and finally meat-eaters in this population had 7.6 per cent prevalence.

The usefulness of vegan diets was eventually endorsed even by the American Diabetes Association when in 2010, their Clinical Practice Guidelines stated that plant-based diets had been shown to improve metabolic control in persons with diabetes (American Diabetes Association, 2010).

DIGESTIVE SYSTEM

What we eat affects our whole body but the digestive system is the first point of contact and thus reacts very strongly to diet.

One of the clearest effects of diet on the digestive system is the composition of gut bacteria (gut microbiome). There are many different species of bacteria that can live in the intestines and diet strongly influences which species thrive and which are suppressed. High fat and high sugar diets are suspected of contributing to growing epidemics of chronic illness, including obesity and inflammatory bowel disease.

David *et al.* (2014) investigated the effect of two distinctly different diets on human gut microbiome. They assigned one group of study participants to a plant-based diet based on grains, pulses, fruits and vegetables; and the second group to an animal-based diet rich in meats, eggs and cheeses. The effects of the diet change after just five days were astonishing. The animal-based diet increased the abundance of bile-tolerant microorganisms that produce many potentially harmful by-products and decreased the levels of bacteria that metabolise plant starches and fibre. The increase in the abundance and activity of the species *Bilophila wadsworthia* on the animal-based diet supports a link between dietary fat, bile acids and changes in gut microbiome capable of triggering inflammatory bowel disease.

Another recent study focused on reviewing available data on vegan, vegetarian and omnivore gut health and, in particular, the type of gut bacteria that these diets promote (Glick-Bauer and Yeh, 2014). The study discovered that the relationship between diet and gut bacteria follows a continuum, with vegan bacterial populations being the most distinct from those of omnivores. The vegan gut microbiome has the highest proportions of health beneficial and protective bacteria. This results in reduced levels of inflammation and may be the key feature linking the vegan diet to its multiple health benefits.

In a small study, six meat-eating obese people with type 2 diabetes and/or high blood pressure were assigned to a strict vegetarian, high-fibre, low-fat diet for one month (Kim *et al.*, 2013). At the end of the month, the diet had not only achieved weight loss but just about every marker of previous bad health – cholesterol, fats and blood sugar – was improved. Two people's results showed they could no longer be diagnosed as diabetics. The diet also positively altered the ratio of gut bacteria

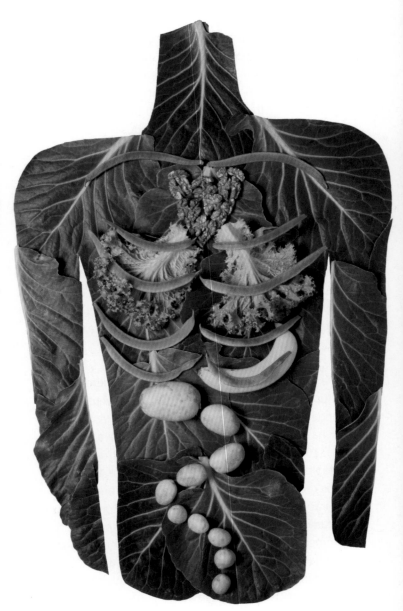

– it encouraged the beneficial bacteria and decreased the numbers of pathogenic bacteria, thus significantly decreasing the level of gut inflammation in the patients.

Chronic gut inflammation is linked to many health issues such as inflammatory bowel disease, metabolic syndrome, immune system disorders and rheumatoid arthritis. It's now clear that a high-fat, high-sugar Western style diet significantly contributes to this scenario and encourages bacteria that produce harmful substances that not only increase inflammation but some of them are also carcinogenic (Huang *et al.*, 2013).

Inflammatory bowel diseases (IBD) are a general term for a group of diseases that affect the intestine. Two common ones are ulcerative colitis (UC) and Crohn's Disease (CD). UC affects mostly the colon whilst CD can occur anywhere along the gastrointestinal tract. Both cause high levels of inflammation, inability to digest or tolerate many types of food and increased permeability of the gut wall compromising the immune system. Huang *et al.* (2013) reviewed the evidence and suggest that a Western diet high in fat and sugars promotes pathogenic bacteria to a degree that causes high inflammation followed by disruption of gut wall integrity in genetically susceptible people. On the other hand, fibre-rich food encourages the growth of bacteria that produce compounds that help lower cholesterol, decrease inflammation and may act as anticarcinogenic agents to protect against colon cancer.

Chiba *et al.* (2015) used a plant-based diet to treat patients with CD. Although their diet does allow some animal products, their research points at fibre and other plant compounds as the nutrients that promote gut health, supress inflammation and act as a substrate for 'good' bacteria. They recommend a plant-based diet for CD for all patients as an essential part of the treatment.

Vegetarian diets have also proved very useful in prevention of diverticular disease (Crowe *et al.*, 2011). In diverticular disease, small bulges or pockets (diverticula) develop in the lining of the intestine. This together with muscle spasms along the diverticula can cause abdominal pain, bloating and other digestive problems. Diverticula can become inflamed or infected causing further issues. In this study, the participants' diets and health were followed for an average of 11.6 years and the observed diet effect was considerable – vegetarians had a 31 per cent lower risk of diverticular disease compared with meat eaters. The association was very strong between high fibre intake and low risk of the disease – people with the highest fibre intakes (more than 26 grams a day) had a 41 per cent lower risk.

Research clearly points at plant-based foods as very beneficial for digestive health whilst it consistently shows that animal-based diets are detrimental. A vegan diet can significantly reduce intestinal inflammation in the general population which can help prevent or treat many conditions. IBD patients may need medication but the right diet can help them heal and stay in remission.

CASE STUDY: MARK GIBSON, UK

Late teens is an important time in social development when dating is the done thing but in my case irritable bowel syndrome (IBS) made me feel really uncomfortable and embarrassed in social settings. When I started work, I had to ask to be excused more than is reasonable. On a night out to the pub I'd constantly be running to the toilet for no reason but IBS. That was my life day in day out.

I became vegetarian at around the age of twenty for moral reasons. The situation remained the same with regards to IBS. I did not receive any medical advice to rectify the problem. My diet was varied – anything as long as it was vegetarian suitable. The constant discomfort made me ask myself what could be the cause? Was it the drink? No, IBS persisted even when I avoided alcohol. Could it be due to stress? I was prone to anxiety, but when I was completely contented in life IBS still persisted. Resignedly, it was something I just had to live with...

...until, at about age 28, I took the logical step for a vegetarian and became vegan. I hadn't reckoned on there being a bonus health benefit in store. However, when I became vegan the irritable bowel syndrome was cured, it stopped completely! There was no regime before as nothing seemed to improve the situation. I still don't have a regime except that I am vegan. I can only conclude therefore, that eliminating dairy from my diet solved the problem of my IBS. I am 37 now and since the day I became vegan approximately ten years ago I have not experienced an irritable bowel, which looking back is quite remarkable.

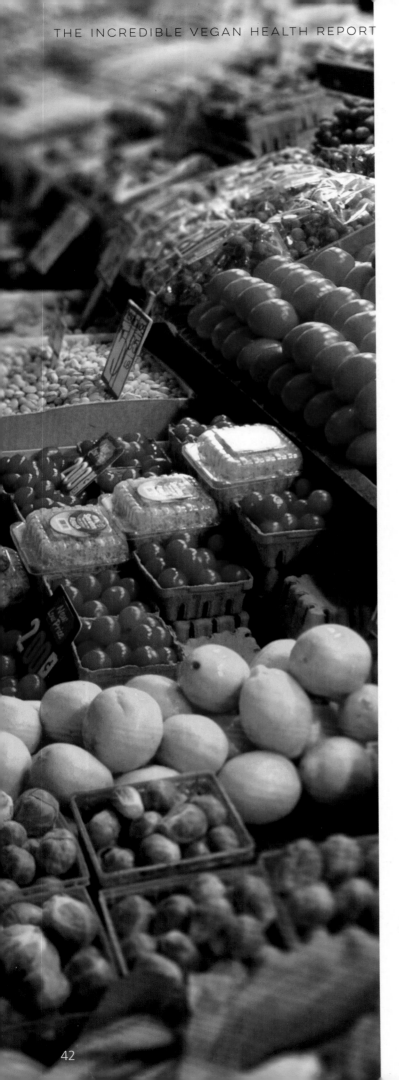

FIBROMYALGIA

Fibromyalgia is a condition characterised by widespread pain, painful response to pressure, morning stiffness, fatigue, sleep disturbances and can include many other health issues. There is no known cause but it has been suggested that central nervous system malfunction leading to amplification of pain is one of the mechanisms. External factors including infection, trauma, stress and toxic substances may also contribute to the development of the disease.

Research suggests a raw vegan diet can improve the condition in general and some symptoms in particular. In a Finnish study a group of fibromyalgia patients were put on a raw vegan diet for three months (Kaartinen et al., 2000). The results revealed significant improvements in pain, joint stiffness, quality of sleep and a significant reduction in weight (most of the patients were overweight) and cholesterol levels.

A similar study was performed in the USA where fibromyalgia patients were put on an almost entirely raw vegan diet for two months (Donaldson et al., 2001). The majority of them responded to the diet with all parameters improving dramatically (physical functioning, bodily pain, general health, vitality, social functioning, emotional and mental health). In those who stayed on the diet for seven months all symptoms except bodily pain subsided to the point that they were undistinguishable from the normal population and the level of pain decreased substantially too.

Lamb et al. (2011) tested the impact of a conventional healthy diet (based on general government guidelines) on fibromyalgia sufferers and compared it with the effects of an elimination diet. The study participants were on either diet for four weeks. The elimination diet excluded seafood, refined and added sugars, artificial colourings, flavourings and sweeteners, caffeinated beverages, gluten-containing grains, eggs and dairy products and foods high in arachidonic acid (many meats and meat products, processed fatty foods). During the elimination diet the patients were also given botanical extracts (high in antioxidants and other phytonutrients).

The conventional diet only mildly improved the symptoms but the elimination diet brought about a significant decrease in both pain and stiffness scores. Participants also had better pain tolerance at five tender points during the elimination diet.

Although research on a purely vegan diet and fibromyalgia is scarce, there is evidence it can be very helpful and alleviate many symptoms with no adverse effects.

KIDNEY HEALTH

The kidneys are affected by diet to a high degree. During digestion, when foods are broken down, absorbed and metabolised they either produce acid or alkali. The main acid forming foods are red and white meat, fish, cheese, eggs, sugar, some grain products and alcohol and the kidneys are worked harder when there is too much acid in the diet. If the diet consistently contains too many acid-producing foods or if the kidneys are damaged and don't function well, it can lead to a condition called metabolic acidosis (which is a constant acid overload of the body that can affect numerous biochemical processes and lead to poorer health and disease).

Most fruit and vegetables are alkali-producers and therefore beneficial for kidney health. Among people with chronic kidney disease (CKD), who have compromised kidney function and need to reduce the amount of acid their diet produces, increasing fruit and vegetable intake has proven to be a highly effective approach (Goraya et al., 2013). A scientific team of experts on kidney health studied dietary acid load and how it affects the kidneys. They found that people with the most acid-producing diets had the highest risk of CKD (Banerjee et al., 2014) and that in people who already have CKD, a diet high in acid-producing foods increases the risk of end stage renal disease (Banerjee et al., 2015).

Research has shown that among people with any degree of kidney damage, consumption of animal protein increases the risk of further kidney deterioration (Knight et al., 2003). And Moe et al. (2011) agree that for patients with CKD, the origin of protein in their diet matters – non-animal protein is more protective whilst animal protein increases markers of kidney damage. This is due to higher phosphorus content of animal protein and higher proportion of sulphur amino acids contributing to more acid.

The lifetime prevalence of kidney stones is around 10 per cent in developed countries (Tourney et al., 2014). The Oxford arm of the comprehensive EPIC study examined the relationship between diet and kidney stones in over 51,000 people in the UK (Tourney et al., 2014). Analyses confirmed that meat and meat products consumption increases the risk – those in the top third of intake had a 64 per cent higher risk compared to those in the bottom third. Data from this study also suggest that diets high in fruit, fibre and magnesium can offer protection against kidney stones. Higher magnesium intakes (plant-based foods are the main sources) can reduce the risk of kidney stones by binding oxalate (the main crystal and stone forming compound). On the other hand, a diet high in animal protein may result in an increased stone risk by producing an acid load that increases urinary calcium and oxalate levels and also produces uric acid (another compound that can form kidney stones).

An earlier study by Borghi et al. (2002) supports these findings. Their conclusion was that for people with recurrent calcium oxalate kidney stones, reducing animal protein and salt intake is crucial for successful treatment.

Heilberg and Goldfarb (2013) reviewed data on diet and kidney stones and reached the conclusion that to prevent and treat kidney stones, a plant-based diet is very important. According to their research this applies to oxalate, purine and cystine stones – for all these animal protein is the main risk factor. They recommended increased intake of fruit and vegetables and wholegrains and an overall vegetarian diet.

A vegan diet with limited acid-producing foods and high in fruits and vegetables can protect the kidneys in many ways and if the kidney function has been compromised, it can help the kidneys recover or minimise further damage. Ströhle et al. (2011) showed that a vegan diet has a virtually neutral acid-alkali balance and can be therefore be very health protective.

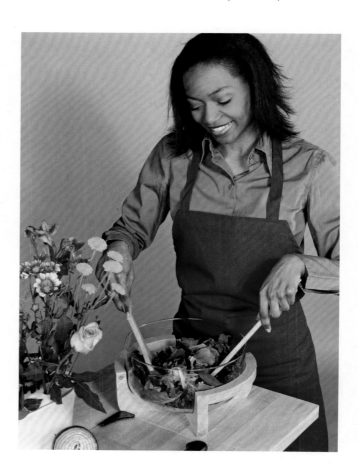

MENTAL HEALTH AND COGNITION

Mental health and cognition are affected by countless factors but in some cases, diet choices can help achieve a difference or lower the risk. A vegan diet that's naturally high in antioxidants, fibre and low in saturated fats seems to be able to lower the risk of cognitive decline and neurodegenerative diseases.

In a study of dietary habits and cognitive function, Eskelinen *et al.* (2011) found that people whose mid-life diets were characterised as healthy (high in plant-based foods, low in saturated fats, etc.) had a decreased risk of dementia and Alzheimer's disease later in life compared with people with unhealthy diets. The difference was staggering – persons who ate the healthiest had an 86-90 per cent decreased risk of dementia and a 90-92 per cent decreased risk of Alzheimer's disease compared with people whose diet was the least healthy.

Another long-term study with a similar design following participants for 20-30 years revealed that people with higher cholesterol levels in mid-life have a significantly higher risk of Alzheimer's disease (1.5 times higher for people with high cholesterol) and dementia (1.5 times higher risk for people with increased cholesterol levels) later in life (Solomon *et al.*, 2009).

Apart from genetic and age-related factors, the risk of Alzheimer's disease is also increased by elevated blood lipids, blood pressure and diabetes. At the International Conference on Nutrition and the Brain in Washington (USA) in 2013, experts in the field were asked to draw and comment on evidence-based guidelines for the prevention of Alzheimer's disease (Barnard *et al.*, 2014). They agreed on the following:

1. Minimise your intake of saturated fats and trans fats. Saturated fat is found primarily in dairy products, meats, and certain oils (coconut and palm oils). Trans fats are found in many snack pastries and fried foods and are listed on labels as "partially hydrogenated oils."

2. Vegetables, legumes (beans, peas, and lentils), fruits and wholegrains should replace meats and dairy products as primary staples of the diet.

3. Vitamin E should come from foods, rather than supplements. Healthful food sources of vitamin E include seeds, nuts, green leafy vegetables, and wholegrains. The recommended dietary allowance (RDA) for vitamin E is 15 mg per day.

4. A reliable source of vitamin B12, such as fortified foods or a supplement providing at least the recommended daily allowance (2.4 mg per day for adults), should be part of your daily diet. Have your blood levels of vitamin B12 checked regularly as many factors, including age, may impair absorption.

5. If using multiple vitamins, choose those without iron and copper and consume iron supplements only when directed by your physician.

6. Although aluminium's role in Alzheimer's disease remains a matter of investigation, those who desire to minimise their exposure can avoid the use of cookware, antacids, baking powder, or other products that contain aluminium.

7. Include aerobic exercise in your routine, equivalent to 40 minutes of brisk walking 3 times per week.

Although it's the diet as a whole that matters, berries in particular have been shown by independent long-term studies to have a protective effect due to their high flavonoid content. Flavonoids are a group of natural compounds found only in plants, they have antioxidant properties and might be neuroprotective. In one of the long-term studies, nearly 130,000 participants were followed for over 20 years. At the end of the study, scientists analysed the data and found that those who consumed the most berries had significantly lower risk of developing Parkinson's disease (Gao *et al.*, 2012). Another study followed over 16,000 people, also for over 20 years, analysed their diets and measured cognitive function (Devore *et al.*, 2012). The results showed that high intake of flavonoids, especially from berries, slowed rates of cognitive decline.

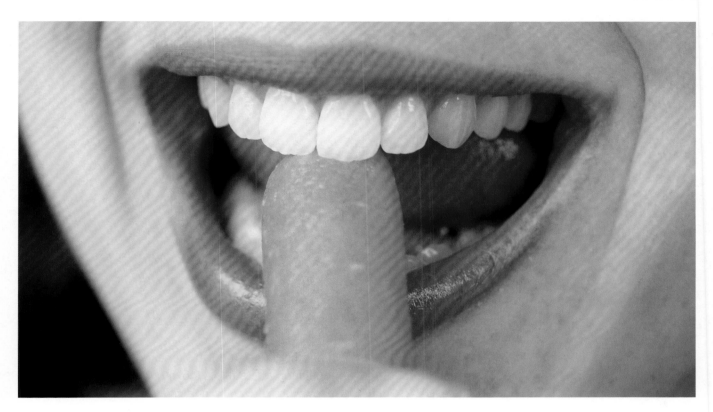

More and more studies are now linking mental and physical health. As illustrated above, many dietary risk factors that can contribute to cardiovascular disease, diabetes and other chronic diseases can also increase the speed of cognitive decline. Although we don't know the precise mechanisms of how exactly the nerve system is affected by diet, we now know that a diet based on plant foods can be protective and reduce the risk of neurodegenerative diseases.

METABOLIC SYNDROME

Metabolic syndrome is a cluster of metabolic risk factors associated with premature death and an increased risk of heart disease and type 2 diabetes. The main symptoms are abdominal obesity, raised fat levels (triglycerides) in the blood, higher blood pressure and higher than normal blood sugar levels.

And not only does metabolic syndrome significantly increase the risk of diabetes and cardiovascular disease but as research shows, it also makes people more prone to cognitive decline and depression. A study of over 7,000 people over the age of 65 revealed that people with metabolic syndrome are at an increased risk of cognitive decline (Raffaitin et al., 2011).

Studies looking at the diets of middle-aged and elderly people of different ethnicities show that vegetarians are at a much lower risk of metabolic syndrome than meat-eaters (Chiang et al., 2013; Gadgil et al., 2014; Rizzo et al., 2011). One of these studies quantified the risk of developing metabolic syndrome which was 54-57 per cent lower for vegetarians (Chiang et al., 2013).

As many studies mentioned above show, vegans tend to have a healthier weight, better blood sugar and fat levels and their digestive system tends to be healthier. Many of these effects are linked to a high consumption of antioxidant and fibre rich foods, mainly fruits and vegetables and wholegrains but research shows other foods contribute to the beneficial effects too. A recent study of over 800 people analysed their diets and assessed their intake of nuts in total, tree nuts (walnuts, almonds, hazelnuts, cashews, pistachios and Brazil nuts) and peanuts (which actually are pulses) (Jaceldo-Siegl et al., 2014). The results showed that people eating the most tree nuts were the least likely to be obese and suffer from metabolic syndrome. Total nut intake among the highest tree nut consumers was 31.6 grams (a good handful) per day.

And another study suggests that eating pulses on a regular basis can prevent metabolic syndrome (Hosseinpour-Niazi et al., 2012). In the study, people who consumed the most pulses (around 2.5 portions per week) had lower blood pressure, blood sugar levels and a healthier blood fat profile than those people who consumed less. Researchers calculated that these people had 75 per cent lower risk of developing the metabolic syndrome.

LONGEVITY AND MORTALITY

Oxidative stress has been implicated in the development of many chronic diseases related to aging such as cancer and cardiovascular disease. The idea is that free radicals (by-products of metabolism) cause oxidative damage to vital molecules in the cells which can lead to disease and faster ageing. Antioxidants from the diet scavenge free radicals and thus help protect the DNA and other molecules. If the diet doesn't provide enough antioxidants, it can lead to the accumulation of unrepaired damage. Unprocessed plant foods are rich sources of antioxidants and therefore vegan diets should

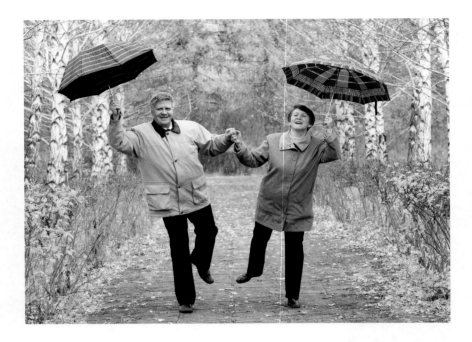

provide the body with a substantial amount. Krajcovicová-Kudlá ková et al. (2008) compared groups of young (20-30 years) and elderly (60-70 years) vegetarian and non-vegetarian women and measured the products of oxidative damage of DNA (DNA strand breaks), lipids and proteins in their blood. They found no significant difference between the two young groups in values of oxidative damage or levels of antioxidant vitamins (C, ß-carotene). However, the older vegetarian group had significantly lower values of DNA and lipid damage and significantly higher levels of antioxidants compared to the older omnivore group. The results suggest that a plant-based diet can limit oxidative damage linked to ageing. The authors also highlighted that based on their previous studies, vegetarian women had significantly higher intake of protective foods (fruit, vegetables, wholegrains, nuts and pulses) than non-vegetarians.

A large review of studies looking into the long-term intake of fruit and vegetables discovered that a higher intake was associated with lower mortality (ie longer life) and cardiovascular mortality in particular (Wang et al., 2014).

As previous chapters demonstrated, vegans have a lower risk of many diseases and have a higher intake of protective plant foods so it follows that their overall longevity should be above the average age. Orlich et al. (2013) investigated dietary patterns and mortality rates in a large American and Canadian population. They found that vegans had 15 per cent lower all-cause mortality compared with meat-eaters.

In another large study, this time of a Spanish population, the authors looked at dietary patterns and many types of food in particular in relation to mortality (Martínez-González et al., 2014). They found that people whose diets contained the most fruit, vegetables, nuts, cereals, pulses, olive oil and potatoes and minimal amounts of animal fats, eggs, fish, dairy products and meats or meat products had significantly lower mortality. In fact, people whose diets were the most plant-based had mortality rates 41 per cent lower than the rest of the population. That means that over the course of the study, people whose diets were mostly vegan were healthier and much fewer of them died compared to the rest of the population.

And finally, the EPIC study that included more than 450,000 participants to study their dietary habits and mortality came to a similar conclusion (Leenders et al., 2014). People consuming more than 570 g of fruits and vegetables a day had lower risks of death from diseases of the circulatory, respiratory and digestive system when compared with participants consuming less than 250 g a day. In more detailed analyses, raw vegetable consumption was showing an even stronger association with lower mortality rates.

Overall, the conclusions these studies reach point in the direction of vegans living longer, healthier lives.

VEGAN ATHLETES

As the number of vegans is growing, so is the number of vegan athletes. A vegan diet can not only meet their nutritional needs but also offer many advantages (Amit, CPS, 2010). Plant-based foods are easier to digest, providing the body with enough energy through carbohydrates, plentiful protein and a wealth of anti-inflammatory antioxidants. As such, vegan diets can help faster recovery and supply easily accessible energy.

Here are a few examples of vegan athletes illustrating the wide range of sports and achievements (for more information and an updated list please see www.greatveganathletes.com):

SCOTT JUREK, USA – ULTRAMARATHON RUNNER, VEGAN SINCE 1997

Scott won Western States 100 mile endurance run seven times, Millwok 100k three times, he was the first American winner of the Spartathon (246k), he also won Leona Divide 50 mile run four times, set ten ultramarathon course records and won at least 24 ultramarathons between 77km and 246km. He became the American record-setter for the 24 hour run in Greece where he ran 165 miles. And in July 2015, he set the world record on the Apalachian trail – in just over 46 days he managed to run 2,189 miles, across 14 states and 515,000 feet of elevation change. He averaged nearly 50 miles a day.

PATRIK BABOUMIAN, GERMANY – GERMANY'S STRONGEST MAN, VEGAN SINCE 2011

He holds the world record for carrying a staggering 550 kilos for a length of over 10 metres. He holds the world log lift record for under 105kg, with a 165kg lift, as well as the German heavyweight log lift record. His heaviest log lift is 190kg. In 2012 he won the German log lift title for the fourth time in a row and set a keg lift world record (115 kg). He took the European Powerlifting title in Finland and in 2012 he competed in the European Powerlifting Championships where he squatted 300kg, bench pressed 200kg and deadlifted 330kg. In 2013 Patrik was invited to compete in the FIBO Champions League against some of the sport's elite and he recorded a win in the crucifix hold.

MAC DANZIG, USA – A MIXED MARTIAL ARTS (MMA) COMPETITOR, VEGAN SINCE 2004

Being actively involved and competing at top levels of Mixed Martial Arts, Mac came across a vegan trainer who aided him in transitioning to a plant-based diet in 2004. In 2005, he won the King Of The Cage Lightweight Championship. He defended the title four times. Later that year Mac entered The Ultimate Fighter 6 competition which he won. Among other achievements, he was awarded Knockout of the Night when he beat Joe Stephenson in December 2010.

BRENDAN BRAZIER, CANADA – IRONMAN TRIATHLETE AND ENDURANCE RUNNER, LONG-TERM VEGAN

Canadian triathlete Brendan Brazier has won triathlons at Olympic distance, Half Ironman and full Ironman, which is a 2.4 mile swim, 112 mile cycle and marathon (26.2 mile) run. He has set the Bigfoot Half Ironman course record twice and was twice Canadian 50k champion. Brendan is a big supporter of a plant-based diet, especially for athletes, and openly speaks about the advantages of this lifestyle as it allows one to train harder and recover faster.

TIM SHIEFF, UK – FREERUNNER AND PARKOUR ATHLETE, VEGAN SINCE 2012

Also known by his freerunning name 'Livewire', Tim Shieff is one of the best known and most successful athletes in freerunning and parkour. In 2014 he completed stage one of the American Ninja Warrior competition in 62 seconds, beating the existing record by ten seconds. He was also captain of team Europe and led the team to victory.

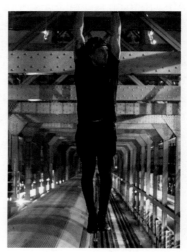

FIONA OAKES, UK – MARATHON RUNNER, LONG-TERM VEGAN

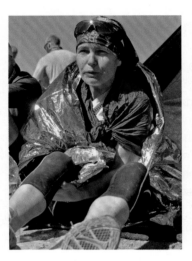

Fiona ran countless marathons in the last 10 years and is also a firefighter. She was previously an award winning cyclist in the UK as well and has won many marathons. In 2013 she ran the North Pole Marathon which she not only completed but also won the women's race, came third to two male competitors and broke the women's course record by an incredible 45 minutes. Later that year she became the fastest woman ever to complete a marathon on all continents. She also set the Guiness world record for the shortest aggregate time for those runs and as part of that marathon series she set the course record for the Antarctic Ice Marathon. In July 2014 she ran the Rio marathon and in doing so broke two of her own Guiness world records. Later that year Fiona ran seven marathons in seven consecutive days and in 2015 she took on the challenge of running a marathon a day for seven days, each on a different continent.

CATHERINE JOHNSON, USA – CYCLOCROSS CHAMPION, VEGAN SINCE 1998

After running several marathons over 1999-2000, Catherine worked as a cycle messenger and started serious cyclocross racing. Highlights include finishing 8th in the Capital Cross Classic 2006 and 6th in the Boulder Short Track Series 2006. She won the Boulder Cyclocross Series in 2005. Catherine retains a passionate determination to excel as a cyclist and is proud of her veganism.

CATRA CORBETT, USA – ULTRAMARATHON RUNNER, LONG-TERM VEGAN

Catra has run over 250 ultramarathons. She holds the womens' record for completing the John Muir Trail twice (out and back), a total of 424 miles, and has the second best all time result for a woman running one way (212 miles). In November 2011 she ran her 80th 100 mile race. In early 2013 she ran her 86th race at 100 miles, the Razorback 100. She finished as the overall winner, beating all male competitors as well as winning the women's race.

STEPH DAVIS, USA – CLIMBER, VEGAN SINCE 2002

Steph made US history for women in the athletic world of rock climbing. She has been the only woman to ever free-climb a number of popular peaks such as Torre Egger in Patagonia in just one day and was the second to free-climb El Capitan in Yosemite National Park in one day. As well as pioneering a number of difficult climbs, Steph has undertaken many challenging base jumps and is an experienced wingsuit flyer.

RUTH HEIDRICH, USA – ENDURANCE ATHLETE, VEGAN SINCE 1982

Ruth was diagnosed with an aggressive breast cancer and turned vegan in 1982, aged 47, in response to the diagnosis. She has won over 900 medals for running of all distances such as the first age-group place in the New Zealand Ironman Triathlon and the Japan Ironman Triathlon in 1988. In 1997 she won the same in the US National Senior Olympics Triathlon and later that year she won the first place in age-group at Hawaii State Senior Olympics in seven seperate track and 10k road races.

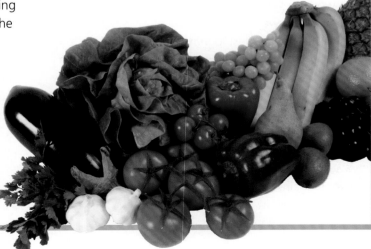

Lanou AJ and Svenson B. 2010. Reduced cancer risk in vegetarians: an analysis of recent reports. *Cancer Management Research*. 3: 1-8.

Le LT and Sabaté J. 2014. Beyond meatless, the health effects of vegan diets: findings from the Adventist cohorts. *Nutrients*. 6 (6) 2131-2147.

Leenders M, Boshuizen HC, Ferrari P et al., 2014. Fruit and vegetable intake and cause-specific mortality in the EPIC study. *European Journal of Epidemiology*. 29 (9) 639-352.

Li WQ, Park Y, Wu JW, Ren JS, Goldstein AM, Taylor PR, Hollenbeck AR, Freedman ND and Abnet CC. 2013. Index-based dietary patterns and risk of esophageal and gastric cancer in a large cohort study. *Clinical Gastroenterology and Hepatology*. 11 (9) 1130-1136.

Li S, Flint A, Pai JK, Forman JP, Hu FB, Willett WC, Rexrode KM, Mukamal KJ and Rimm EB. 2014a. Dietary fiber intake and mortality among survivors of myocardial infarction: prospective cohort study. *BMJ*. 348: g2659.

Li S, Flint A, Pai JK, Forman JP, Hu FB, Willett WC, Rexrode KM, Mukamal KJ and Rimm EB. 2014b. Low carbohydrate diet from plant or animal sources and mortality among myocardial infarction survivors. *Journal of the American Heart Association*. 3 (5) e001169.

Liu SZ, Chen WQ, Wang N, Yin MM, Sun XB and He YT. 2014. Dietary factors and risk of pancreatic cancer: a multi-centre case-control study in China. *Asian Pacific Journal of Cancer Prevention*. 15 (18) 7947-7950.

Liu E, McKeown NM, Newby PK, Meigs JB, Vasan RS, Quatromoni PA, D'Agostino RB and Jacques PF. 2009. Cross-sectional association of dietary patterns with insulin-resistant phenotypes among adults without diabetes in the Framingham Offspring Study. *The British Journal of Nutrition*. 102 (4) 576-583.

Lucenteforte E, Garavello W, Bosetti C and La Vecchia C. 2009. Dietary factors and oral and pharyngeal cancer risk. *Oral Oncology*. 45 (6) 461-467.

Mangels AR and Messina V. 2001. Considerations in planning vegan diets: infants. *Journal of the American Dietetic Association*. 101 (6) 670-677.

Martin JM, Trink B, Daneman D, Dosch H-M and Robinson B. 1991. Milk proteins in the etiology of Insulin-Dependent Diabetes mellitus (IDDM). *Annals of medicine*. 23 (4) 447 – 52

Martínez-González MA, Sánchez-Tainta A, Corella D et al. PREDIMED Group. 2014. A provegetarian food pattern and reduction in total mortality in the Prevención con Dieta Mediterránea (PREDIMED) study. *American Journal of Clinical Nutrition*. 100 Suppl 1:320S-328S.

McDougall J, Bruce B, Spiller G, Westerdahl J and McDougall M. 2002. Effects of a very low-fat, vegan diet in subjects with rheumatoid arthritis. *Journal of Alternative and Complementary Medicine*. 8 (1) 71-75.

McDougall J, Thomas LE, McDougall C, Moloney G, Saul B, Finnell JS, Richardson K and Petersen KM. 2014. Effects of 7 days on an ad libitum low-fat vegan diet: the McDougall Program cohort. *Nutrition Journal*. 13: 99.

Melnik BC, John SM and Schmitz G. Over-stimulation of insulin/IGF-1 signaling by western diet may promote diseases of civilization: lessons learnt from laron syndrome. *Nutrition & Metabolism (London)*. 8: 41.

Messina V and Mangels AR. 2001. Considerations in planning vegan diets: children. *Journal of the American Dietetic Association*. 101 (6) 661-669.

Mishra S, Xu J, Agarwal U, Gonzales J, Levin S and Barnard ND. 2013. A multicenter randomized controlled trial of a plant-based nutrition program to reduce body weight and cardiovascular risk in the corporate setting: the GEICO study. *European Journal of Clinical Nutrition*. 67 (7) 718-724.

Moe SM, Zidehsarai MP, Chambers MA, Jackman LA, Radcliffe JS, Trevino LL, Donahue SE and Asplin JR. 2011. Vegetarian compared with meat dietary protein source and phosphorus homeostasis in chronic kidney disease. *Clinical Journal of the American Society of Nephrology*. 6 (2) 257-264.

Morino K, Petersen KF and Shulman GI. 2006. Molecular mechanisms of insulin resistance in humans and their potential links with mitochondrial dysfunction. *Diabetes*. 55 (Suppl. 2) S9-S15.

Müller H, de Toledo FW and Resch KL. 2001. Fasting followed by vegetarian diet in patients with rheumatoid arthritis: a systematic review. *Scandinavian Journal of Rheumatology*. 30 (1) 1-10.

Muntoni S, Cocco P, Aru G and Cucca F. 2000. Nutritional factors and worldwide incidence of childhood type 1 diabetes. *American Journal of Clinical Nutrition*. 71 (6) 1525-1529.

Murphy N, Norat T, Ferrari P, Jenab M et al. 2012. Dietary fibre intake and risks of cancers of the colon and rectum in the European prospective investigation into cancer and nutrition (EPIC). *PLoS One*. 7 (6) e39361.

Nagel G, Weinmayr G, Kleiner A, Garcia-Marcos L, Strachan DP; ISAAC Phase Two Study Group. 2010. Effect of diet on asthma and allergic sensitisation in the International Study on Allergies and Asthma in Childhood (ISAAC) Phase Two. *Thorax*. 65 (6) 516-522.

Nechuta SJ, Caan BJ, Chen WY, Lu W, Chen Z, Kwan ML, Flatt SW, Zheng Y, Zheng W, Pierce JP and Shu XO. 2012. Soy food intake after diagnosis of breast cancer and survival: an in-depth analysis of combined evidence from cohort studies of US and Chinese women. *American Journal of Clinical Nutrition*. 96 (1) 123-132.

Nenonen MT, Helve TA, Rauma AL and Hänninen OO. 1998. Uncooked, lactobacilli-rich, vegan food and rheumatoid arthritis. *British Journal of Rheumatology*. 37 (3) 274-281.

Newby PK, Tucker KL and Wolk A. 2005. Risk of overweight and obesity among semivegetarian, lactovegetarian, and vegan women. *American Journal of Clinical Nutrition*. 81 (6) 1267-1274.

O'Keefe SJ, Li JV, Lahti L, Ou J et al. 2015. Fat, fibre and cancer risk in African Americans and rural Africans. *Nature Communications*. 6:6342.

Ollberding NJ, Lim U, Wilkens LR, Setiawan VW, Shvetsov YB, Henderson BE, Kolonel LN and Goodman MT. 2012. Legume, Soy, Tofu, and Isoflavone Intake and Endometrial Cancer Risk in Postmenopausal Women in the Multiethnic Cohort Study. *Journal of the National Cancer Institute*. 104 (1) 67-76.

Orlich MJ, Singh PN, Sabaté J, Jaceldo-Siegl K, Fan J, Knutsen S, Beeson WL and Fraser GE. 2013. Vegetarian dietary patterns and mortality in Adventist Health Study 2. *JAMA Internal Medicine*. 173 (13) 1230-1238.

Orlich MJ, Jaceldo-Siegl K, Sabaté J, Fan J, Singh PN and Fraser GE. 2014. Patterns of food consumption among vegetarians and non-vegetarians. *British Journal of Nutrition*. 112 (10) 1644-1653.

Ornish D, Scherwitz LW, Billings JH, Brown SE, Gould KL, Merritt TA, Sparler S, Armstrong WT, Ports TA, Kirkeeide RL, Hogeboom C and Brand RJ. 1998. Intensive lifestyle changes for reversal of coronary heart disease. *JAMA*. 280 (23) 2001-2007.

Ornish D, Weidner G, Fair WR et al. 2005. Intensive lifestyle changes may affect the progression of prostate cancer. *Journal of Urology*. 174 (3) 1065-1070.

Ornish D, Magbanua MJ, Weidner G, Weinberg V, Kemp C, Green C, Mattie MD, Marlin R, Simko J, Shinohara K, Haqq CM and Carroll PR. 2008. Changes in prostate gene expression in men undergoing an intensive nutrition and lifestyle intervention. *Proceedings of the National Academy of Sciences of the USA*. 105 (24) 8369-8374.

Palladino-Davis AG, Mendez BM, Fisichella PM and Davis CS. Dietary habits and esophageal cancer. *Diseases of the Esophagus*. 28 (1) 59-67.

Pan SY, Ugnat AM, Mao Y, Wen SW, Johnson KC; Canadian Cancer Registries Epidemiology Research Group. 2004. A case-control study of diet and the risk of ovarian cancer. *Cancer Epidemiology, Biomarkers & Prevention*. 13 (9) 1521-1527.

Papaioannou MD, Koufaris C and Gooderham NJ. 2014. The cooked meat-derived mammary carcinogen 2-amino-1-methyl-6-phenylimidazo[4,5-b]pyridine (PhIP) elicits estrogenic-like microRNA responses in breast cancer cells. *Toxicology Letters*. 229 (1) 9-16.

Paronen J, Knip M, Savilahti E, Virtanen SM, Ilonen J, Akerblom HK and Vaarala O. 2000. Effect of cow's milk exposure and maternal type 1 diabetes on cellular and humoral immunization to dietary insulin in infants at genetic risk for type 1 diabetes. Finnish Trial to Reduce IDDM in the Genetically at Risk Study Group. *Diabetes*. 49 (10) 1657-1665.

Pastor-Valero M. 2013. Fruit and vegetable intake and vitamins C and E are associated with a reduced prevalence of cataract in a Spanish Mediterranean population. *BMC Ophthalmology*. 13: 52.

Peltonen R, Nenonen M, Helve T, Hänninen O, Toivanen P and Eerola E. 1997. Faecal microbial flora and disease activity in rheumatoid arthritis during a vegan diet. *British Journal of Rheumatology*. 36 (1) 64-68.

Perez-Bravo F, Carrasco E, Gutierrez-Lopez MD, Martinez MT, Lopez G and de los Rios MG. 1996. Genetic predisposition and environmental factors leading to the development of insulin-dependent diabetes mellitus in Chilean children. *Journal of Molecular Medicine*. 74 (2) 105-109.

Petersen KF, Dufour S, Befroy D, Garcia R and Shulman GI. 2004. Impaired mitochondrial activity in the insulin-resistant offspring of patients with type 2 diabetes. *New England Journal of Medicine*. 350 (7) 664-671.

Pettersen BJ, Anousheh R, Fan J, Jaceldo-Siegl K and Fraser GE. 2012. Vegetarian diets and blood pressure among white subjects: results from the Adventist Health Study-2 (AHS-2). *Public Health Nutrition*. 15 (10) 1909-1916.

Phillips DI, Caddy S, Ilic V, Fielding BA, Frayn KN, Borthwick AC and Taylor R. 1996. Intramuscular triglyceride and muscle insulin sensitivity: evidence for a relationship in nondiabetic subjects. *Metabolism*. 45 (8) 947–950.

Phillips F; British Nutrition Foundation. 2005. BRIEFING PAPER: Vegetarian nutrition. *Nutrition Bulletin*. 30: 132–167.

Piyathilake CJ, Badiga S, Kabagambe EK, Azuero A, Alvarez RD, Johanning GL, Partridge EE. 2012. A dietary pattern associated with LINE-1 methylation alters the risk of developing cervical intraepithelial neoplasia. *Cancer Prevention Research*. 5 (3) 385-392.

Plant J. 2007. *Your life in your hands, understanding, preventing and overcoming breast cancer*. London: Virgin Publishing Limited.

Public Health England & Food Standards Agency, 2014. National Diet and Nutrition Survey: results from Years 1 to 4 (combined) of the rolling programme for 2008 and 2009 to 2011 and 2012.

Raffaitin C, Féart C, Le Goff M, Amieva H, Helmer C, Akbaraly TN, Tzourio C, Gin H and Barberger-Gateau P. 2011. Metabolic syndrome and cognitive decline in French elders: The Three-City Study. *Neurology*. 76 (6) 518-525.

Rizzo NS, Sabaté J, Jaceldo-Siegl K and Fraser GE. 2011. Vegetarian Dietary Patterns Are Associated With a Lower Risk of Metabolic Syndrome. *Diabetes Care*. 34 (5) 1225-1227.

Rizzo NS, Jaceldo-Siegl K, Sabate J, Fraser GE. 2013. Nutrient profiles of vegetarian and nonvegetarian dietary patterns. *Journal of the Academy of Nutrition and Dietetics*. 113 (12) 1610-1619.

Rodríguez-Rodríguez E, Perea JM, Jiménez AI, Rodríguez-Rodríguez P, López-Sobaler AM and Ortega RM. Fat intake and asthma in Spanish schoolchildren. *European Journal of Clinical Nutrition*. 64 (10) 1065-1071.

Sabaté J and Wien M. 2010. Vegetarian diets and childhood obesity prevention. *American Journal of Clinical Nutrition*. 91(5): 1525S–1529S.

Sellmeyer DE, Stone KL, Sebastian A and Cummings SR. 2001. A high ratio of dietary animal to vegetable protein increases the rate of bone loss and the risk of fracture in postmenopausal women. Study of Osteoporotic Fractures Research Group. *American Journal of Clinical Nutrition*. 73 (1) 118-122.

Seyedrezazadeh E, Moghaddam MP, Ansarin K, Vafa MR, Sharma S and Kolahdooz F. 2014. Fruit and vegetable intake and risk of wheezing and asthma: a systematic review and meta-analysis. *Nutrition Reviews*. 72 (7): 411-428.

Shaheen SO, Jameson KA, Syddall HE, Aihie Sayer A, Dennison EM, Cooper C, Robinson SM; Hertfordshire Cohort Study Group. 2010. The relationship of dietary patterns with adult lung function and COPD. *European Respiratory Journal*. 36 (2) 277-284.

Shu XO, Jin F, Dai Q, Wen W, Potter JD, Kushi LH, Ruan Z, Gao YT and Zheng W. 2001. Soyfood intake during adolescence and subsequent risk of breast cancer among Chinese women. *Cancer Epidemiology, Biomarkers & Prevention*. 10(5):483-488.

Shu XO, Zheng Y, Cai H, Gu K, Chen Z, Zheng W and Lu W. 2009. Soy food intake and breast cancer survival. *JAMA*. 302 (22) 2437-2443.

Shu L, Wang XQ, Wang SF, Wang S, Mu M, Zhao Y, Sheng J and Tao FB. Dietary patterns and stomach cancer: a meta-analysis. *Nutrition and Cancer*. 65 (8):1105-1115.

Sieri S, Krogh V, Pala V, Muti P, Micheli A, Evangelista A, Tagliabue G and Berrino F. 2004. Dietary patterns and risk of breast cancer in the ORDET cohort. *Cancer Epidemiology, Biomarkers & Prevention*. 13 (4) 567-572.

Solomon A, Kivipelto M, Wolozin B, Zhou J and Whitmer RA. 2009. Midlife serum cholesterol and increased risk of Alzheimer's and vascular dementia three decades later. *Dementia and Geriatric Cognitive Disorders*. 28 (1) 75-80.

Sparks LM, Xie H, Koza RA, Mynatt R, Hulver MW, Bray GA and Smith SR. 2005. A high-fat diet coordinately downregulates genes required for mitochondrial oxidative phosphorylation in skeletal muscle. *Diabetes*. 54 (7) 1926-1933.

Ströhle A, Waldmann A, Koschizke J, Leitzmann C and Hahn A. 2011. Diet-dependent net endogenous acid load of vegan diets in relation to food groups and bone health-related nutrients: results from the German Vegan Study. *Annals of Nutrition and Metabolism*. 59 (2-4)117-126.

Tantamango-Bartley Y, Jaceldo-Siegl K, Fan J and Fraser G. 2013. Vegetarian diets and the incidence of cancer in a low-risk population. *Cancer Epidemiology, Biomarkers & Prevention*. 22 (2) 286-294.

Tonstad S, Butler T, Yan R and Fraser GE. 2009. Type of vegetarian diet, body weight, and prevalence of type 2 diabetes. *Diabetes Care*. 32 (5) 791-796.

Torfadottir JE, Steingrimsdottir L, Mucci L, Aspelund T, Kasperzyk JL, Olafsson O, Fall K, Tryggvadottir L, Harris TB, Launer L, Jonsson E, Tulinius H, Stampfer M, Adami HO, Gudnason V and Valdimarsdottir UA. 2012. Milk Intake in Early Life and Risk of Advanced Prostate Cancer. *American Journal of Epidemiology*.175 (2) 144-153.

Turney BW, Appleby PN, Reynard JM, Noble JG, Key TJ and Allen NE. 2014. Diet and risk of kidney stones in the Oxford cohort of the European Prospective Investigation into Cancer and Nutrition (EPIC). *European Journal of Epidemiology*. 29 (5) 363-369.

Trepanowski JF and Varady KA. 2015. Veganism Is a Viable Alternative to Conventional Diet Therapy for Improving Blood Lipids and Glycemic Control. *Critical Reviews in Food Science and Nutrition*. 55 (14) 2004-2013.

Tsunehara CH, Leonetti DL and Fujimoto WY. 1990. Diet of second generation Japanese American men with and without non-insulin-dependent diabetes. *American Journal of Clinical Nutrition*. 52: 731-8

Turner-McGrievy GM, Barnard ND, Cohen J, Jenkins DJ, Gloede L and Green AA. 2008. Changes in nutrient intake and dietary quality among participants with type 2 diabetes following a low-fat vegan diet or a conventional diabetes diet for 22 weeks. *Journal of the American Dietetic Association*. 108 (10) 1636-1645.

Turner-McGrievy GM, Davidson CR, Wingard EE, Wilcox S and Frongillo EA. 2015. Comparative effectiveness of plant-based diets for weight loss: a randomized controlled trial of five different diets. *Nutrition*. 31 (2) 350-358.

Tuso PJ, Ismail MH, Ha BP and Bartolotto C. 2013. Nutritional update for physicians: plant-based diets. *Permanente Journal*. 17 (2) 61-66.